Special Praise for *Mind-Body Health and Healing*

"*Mind-Body Health and Healing* is filled with insight and guidance on improving one's life by reducing and avoiding the ravages of stress. Although this long-held concept has produced vast research literature, Dr. Goliszek successfully melds his scientist's skill at investigating complex technical information with a professor's capacity to interpret and instruct. First, he explains the neurobiology and physiology that connect mind and body. Then, he shows how every aspect of our lives—how we think, how we feel about ourselves, the decisions we make, our nutrition and diet, our physical activities, and our faith— affects our attitudes and our health, including how we age. This scholarly work is at once informative, useful, and easy to read."

J. Charles Eldridge, PhD
Professor of Physiology & Pharmacology
Wake Forest University School of Medicine

"Dr. Goliszek's book is the most comprehensive book about the mind-body connection that I've read! It is scientifically based, yet easy to understand. Whether you are a lay person seeking to learn the benefits of various integrative practices and how they work, or a professional looking for a detailed overview with depth, you will find this book an excellent resource guide. The included self-help quizzes and exercises move the reader from a place of observation to engagement. In short, this book is not just about healing, for the serious reader, it is healing."

Sandy Seeber, LPC
President, All My Relations, PA
Co-Owner and Partner, Three Treasures Tai Chi LLC
Winston-Salem, NC

MIND-BODY HEALTH AND HEALING

Mind-Body Health and Healing

Using the Power of the Brain to Prevent Disease, Reduce Stress, and Slow Aging

Andrew Goliszek

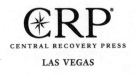

CENTRAL RECOVERY PRESS

LAS VEGAS

Central Recovery Press (CRP) is committed to publishing exceptional materials addressing addiction treatment, recovery, and behavioral healthcare topics, including original and quality books, audio/visual communications, and web-based new media. Through a diverse selection of titles, we seek to contribute a broad range of unique resources for professionals, recovering individuals and their families, and the general public.

For more information, visit www.centralrecoverypress.com.

Publisher: Central Recovery Press
3321 N. Buffalo Drive
Las Vegas, NV 89129

19 18 17 16 15 14   1 2 3 4 5

ISBN: 978-1-937612-73-3 (trade paper)
978-1-937612-74-0 (e-book)

Publisher's Note: This book contains general information about the mind-body connection and utilizing it to heal, and to optimize physical, mental, and emotional health. The information is not medical advice, and should not be treated as such. Central Recovery Press makes no representations or warranties in relation to the medical information in this book; this book is not an alternative to medical advice from your doctor or other professional healthcare provider. If you have any specific questions about any medical matter you should consult your doctor or other professional healthcare provider. If you think you or someone close to you may be suffering from any medical condition, you should seek immediate medical attention. You should never delay seeking medical advice, disregard medical advice, or discontinue medical treatment because of information in this or any book.

Central Recovery Press books represent the experiences of their authors only. Every effort has been made to ensure that events, institutions, and statistics presented in our books as facts are accurate and up-to-date.

Author photo used with permission. ©Lifetouch, Inc.

Cover design and interior design and layout by Sara Streifel, Think Creative Design

TO MY WIFE, KATHY

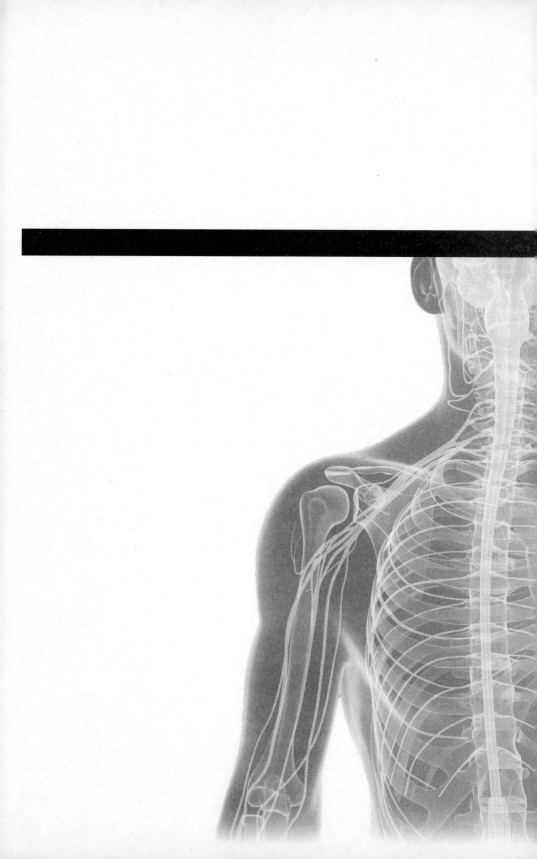

Table of Contents

CHAPTER THREE Using the Mind-Body Connection to Prevent Disease

CHAPTER FOUR Conditioning the Brain to Prevent Illness

CHAPTER FIVE Stress, Mental Health, and the Mind-Body Connection

CHAPTER ELEVEN The Mind-Body Connection in Children and Adolescents

APPENDIX A Time Management and Stress

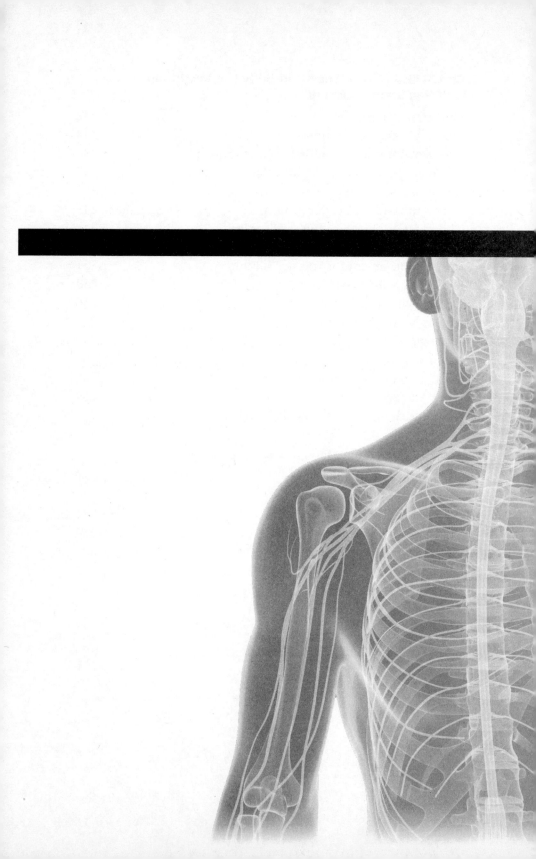

Acknowledgments

A book like this is not possible without the input and expertise of researchers and healthcare professionals who spend their lives helping us learn more about the connection between the mind and body. I would like to thank my former colleagues at Wake Forest University School of Medicine, and particularly Dr. Joan Robinson and Dr. William Sonntag, who mentored me during my early years and helped guide me in my research.

Introduction

As researchers continually discover more about the amazing extent to which the brain has power over the body and may even control healing, we continually marvel at what has become known as the mind-body connection. The premise of this book is that by using a variety of simple techniques and tools we can harness and direct that power for optimum physical, emotional, and behavioral health. These include diet, exercise, attitude adjustment, and, perhaps most importantly, stress reduction.

Mind-body specialists posit that the mind and body are essentially inseparable—that the brain and peripheral nervous system, the endocrine and immune systems, all of our organs and all of our emotional responses, are in constant communication with one another through a common chemical language. Indeed, many of our most deeply felt emotions may be considered by some simply as chemical reactions that take place in the brain and manifest in the body as the states we recognize as love or hate.

Mental states can be fully conscious or unconscious. We can have emotional reactions to situations without being aware of why we are reacting (think "triggers," or "having one's 'buttons' pushed"). Each mental state has a physiology associated with it—a positive or negative effect felt in the physical body. And so, many mind-body therapies focus on becoming more conscious of mental states and using this increased awareness to guide our mental states in a better, less destructive direction.

Scientific studies show that severe prolonged stress and chronic negative thinking can compromise the immune system, laying the groundwork for disease to take hold. One way that many mind-body therapies work is by reducing stress. So it is helpful to understand what stress is and the role it plays in health and well-being.

Studies have also revealed that individuals with a positive attitude toward life tend to become sick less often than those with a negative attitude.

Even though these concepts may be new to you, studies in the mind-body connection are showing us that our minds play a major role in influencing our level of wellness. By using the simple techniques I outline in this book to condition your brain, you will be able to harness and direct your own brain power to boost immunity and effect healing.

It is my hope that after reading this book, you'll be better equipped to take charge of your mind as well as your body and condition yourself to remain healthy throughout life.

> The mind-body concept is defined as the interaction that takes place among our thoughts, our body, and our external world. A new science that studies this link is called psychoneuroimmunology (PNI). PNI describes ways in which our emotions and attitude, both positive and negative, can affect our health and also the outcome of medical treatment.

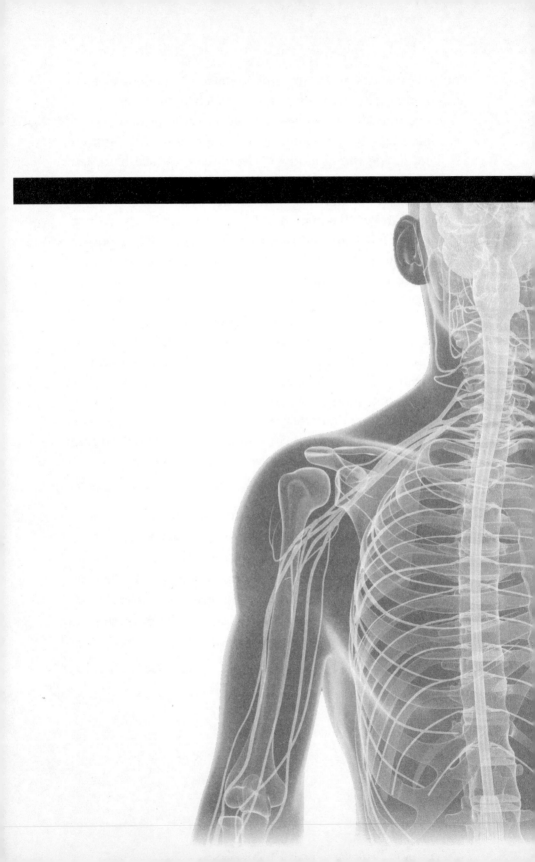

CHAPTER ONE

The Brain: Where It All Starts

Psychologists, philosophers, researchers, and others postulate that it is the physical brain that creates, or gives rise to, the ephemeral mind. This is in contrast to the ancients, who thought that the heart was the seat, not only of emotion, but thinking as well. It's important to note that the mind is not synonymous with the brain. Instead, in our definition, the mind consists of mental states that include thoughts, emotions, beliefs, attitudes, and images. The brain is the hardware that allows us to experience these mental states.

The human brain is an exceedingly complex and marvelous organ comprising a network of neural connections and approximately 100 billion nerve cells known as neurons.

But the human brain is much more than a collection of neurons. If that's all it were, we wouldn't be nearly as smart as an octopus, the brain of which can have as many as 150 billion neurons. And if numbers of neurons were the criterion, we certainly would not be as intelligent as dolphins, elephants, or sperm whales, the latter having brains almost five times the size of ours. Weighing in at a mere 2 percent of our total body weight, the human brain is one of the marvels of evolution.

Within its many folds is an organic computer that rivals anything we may have on our desktop. It was the human brain, after all, that invented the computer.

Why should we be surprised, then, that when we consciously tap into that brainpower, we can use one of the greatest forces of nature to regulate the life processes that keep us healthy and disease-free? The interplay between the physical brain and the intangible mind is manifest in the interaction of the physical body and the mental aspects of health and disease. The health of the mind affects the body and the health of the body affects the mind.

The Brain Creates the Mind

The brain is the physical organ that gives rise to the mind, which in turn is the thinking and perceiving part of our consciousness. Our brains are like two-pound computers with empty files, ready to input data as fast as possible. Neural (nerve) connections sprout; and the more we're stimulated and the more data we input during the first few years of our life, the more effectively those connections grow.

During the first ten years of life, the brain's outer portion or cerebral cortex grows the most rapidly and undergoes the greatest amount of change. Therefore, a large amount of sensory input and education is essential for proper growth, development, learning, and memory. While the expression "use it or lose it," is true at all ages when it comes to the brain, it's especially true at this critical time of life. Children who are not held, cuddled, or adequately stimulated during infancy will not fully develop emotionally. At the other end of the age spectrum, older individuals who no longer perform regular mental activities will have increased memory loss and a decreased capacity in certain intellectual skills.

Throughout our lives, we're constantly using our brain—both consciously and subconsciously—for a variety of functions, even during sleep. The old adage that we only use 10 percent of our brain is not true.

On the other hand, the mind refers to the collection of experiences, memories, feelings, and emotions that, together with our subconscious, make us who we are. The mind-body connection is sometimes called the brain-body connection because our brain is really the control center for every one of our organ systems and the catalyst that triggers the multitude of chemical reactions that control our lives from before birth until we take our last breath (at least).

We don't fully understand the intricacies of how nerve networks operate, but we do know that the brain has an incredible ability to change connections in response to sensory stimuli. This ability is called neuroplasticity and is responsible for creating feelings and emotions and producing cognitive behaviors such as thinking and memory that change with our life experiences. Until recently, we didn't realize the extent to which we're consciously able to trigger the brain—with no external stimuli at all —into actions that can literally alter the thousands of biochemical reactions occurring in our bodies every second.

For example, visualization or imaging is being used along with traditional chemotherapy treatment to help patients destroy malignant cells. Prayer sessions are becoming a part of healthcare at many hospitals owing to the belief (supported by some research) that spirituality plays a vital role in a patient's healing process. Both imaging and prayer are examples of how the brain, as a result of stimulation by our thoughts, can be mobilized to boost the immune system enough to influence diseases as life-threatening as heart disease and cancer.

The Brain and Immunity

Development of the immune system begins during the first few weeks after conception. Neural folds appear and release cells that form what is known as the neural crest. The neural crest then contributes to the proper formation of the thymus gland, which is necessary for the full and effective development of the immune system. Once the central nervous system (CNS)—consisting of the brain and spinal cord—develops, it begins to communicate with the immune system to create immune responses.

Individuals with poor brain development, or with psychiatric and neurological disorders, often have poor immune responsiveness, lowered antibody production, and impaired lymphocyte activity. Some of these individuals, particularly those suffering with psychiatric disorders, can be helped with the techniques described in this book. The sensitivity of the CNS is one reason prenatal care is so important. Unless the CNS develops and grows properly in an environment without toxins such as alcohol, nicotine, drugs, and other agents, the immune system will not develop properly either. Babies are then born who may have underdeveloped spleens, thymuses, and lymph nodes, with a subsequent decrease in white blood cell production. Many children whose mothers may not have known they were pregnant until the second or third month are born much more susceptible to infections and diseases.

The nervous system is the first system to be visible during early embryonic development. Once it begins to form, everything else follows. The endocrine and lymphatic organs, together with the brain and nerves, form the neuro-endocrine-immune system, which controls the healing process and keeps us healthy. Some of the brain's structures, such as the hypothalamus and pituitary, play an especially critical role in our ability to respond to events happening around us. The manner in which we respond, however, is the result of brain conditioning, much like the conditioning of our muscles during physical exercise or training.

Figure 1.1: Main Components of the Developed Brain

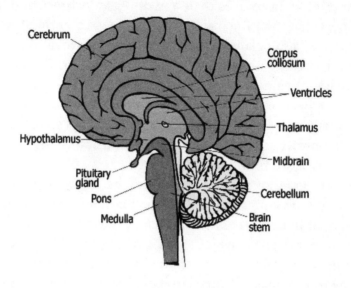

Hypothalamus/Pituitary: The Brain's Thermostat

The lower area of the brain contains a section called the hypothalamus. Known as the body's thermostat, the hypothalamus maintains homeostasis, the constant state in which our body operates. Functions such as heart rate, blood pressure, body temperature, growth, metabolism, electrolyte balance, hunger, sleep, wakefulness, and breathing are controlled by signals generated by this area of the brain.

In order to function properly and direct the brain, the hypothalamus receives signals from the skin, eyes, nose, peripheral nerves, and the multitude of internal receptors that respond to changes in temperature, fluid concentration, and pressure. Because it's so sensitive to stressors and environmental signals, the hypothalamus is also involved in an immense number of biochemical reactions, and is the reason why stress can have such a deleterious effect on so many different organ systems. Altering the hypothalamus surgically, for example, can literally destroy the immune response.

Directly below the hypothalamus is the pituitary, which releases more hormones than any other endocrine gland. But although it's the principal gland that releases hormones (it's called the master gland of the body), the pituitary cannot do so without chemicals produced by the hypothalamus. The anterior pituitary is involved in many of the reactions occurring during stress, anxiety, and physical trauma. A pathway comprising the hypothalamus, pituitary, and adrenal gland plays an important role in how we deal with both physical and emotional stressors and is discussed in the next chapter.

The posterior pituitary releases two hormones, one of which, vasopressin or antidiuretic hormone (ADH), is important in regulating the body's fluid balance. During stress, it also contributes to the release of cortisol, which depresses the immune system and makes us more prone to illness and disease. In the case of major depression, both vasopressin and cortisol levels are very high. Oxytocin, the other posterior pituitary hormone, is mainly involved in muscle contractions, especially the uterine muscles during the final stages of pregnancy and the mammary gland cells during suckling in order to eject milk. In males, oxytocin increases contractions of the prostate gland and the vas deferens, the vessel that transports sperm.

Recently, a team of scientists from Heptares Therapeutics, a medical company in Hertfordshire, England, discovered the structure of what has been called the brain's "misery molecule." According to the scientists, CRF-1, a protein found in the brain and pituitary cells, triggers the release of stress hormones and may actually contribute to our feelings of stress, anxiety, and even depression. Chief scientific officer Fiona Marshall said that "Stress-related diseases such as depression and anxiety affect a quarter of adults each year, but what many people don't realize is that these conditions are controlled by proteins in the brain, one of which is CRF-1 found in structure of class B GPCR corticotrophin-releasing factor receptor 1." The team soon hopes to develop drugs that can block CRF-1 and blunt the release of chemicals responsible for stress reactions.[1]

The Limbic System

A network of nerves above the hypothalamus, the limbic system is often referred to as the emotional brain. It has a large number of sensory receptors and the greatest concentration of the brain's opiate receptors. The rush or feeling of euphoria one gets after taking an opiate such as heroin or morphine is caused by the binding of such drugs to these opiate receptors.

The limbic system controls and regulates emotions such as fear, rage, love, hate, sexual arousal, aggression, pleasure, and pain. Located here are the so-called punishment and reward centers, believed to be important in learning and in triggering the motivational systems behind behavior that seeks to avoid pain and pursue pleasure. Different areas of this system elicit different responses. Some years ago, I worked with a research scientist who was investigating how tobacco additives could be used to stimulate the areas of the limbic system that produce pleasure responses.

One part of the limbic system important in learning and memory is the hippocampus. Whenever we learn something new, structural changes occur that allow us to remember. New evidence from Alzheimer's patients shows that there is considerable atrophy of the hippocampus, which would explain the loss of memory and the inability to recognize even recent experiences. Neuroplasticity is essentially lost, and the brain can no longer file away information.

It's also believed that the limbic system is the part of the brain most involved with violent behavior. For example, as part of a classic medical experiment, a woman had an electrode inserted in one section of her limbic system and received a mild current. She immediately became angry and violent. When the current was switched off, she again became pleasant and cooperative. There's agreement among neuroscientists that disruption of nerve impulses within the limbic system may be responsible for at least some cases of violent behavior.

Like all other areas of the brain, the limbic system is affected by a number of external signals from the environment, as well as by internal signals we send to ourselves because of the way we think and how we perceive events. No organ is more prone to suggestions than is the brain; and no organ in the human body is more responsive to how the body responds to those suggestions. Fighting a cold or eliminating a tumor often depends in part on the positive signals we send, which in turn unleash a wave of chemicals that trigger the massive immune response that stops disease in its tracks.

Why Placebos Are Effective

In research studies, nearly one-third of patients given nothing more than a placebo—often a sugar pill or a distilled water and salt solution—improve their condition. Why? Obviously something powerful takes place in the brain of the patient. As Dr. Robert DeLap, then head of the US Food and Drug Administration's (FDA) Offices of Drug Evaluation explained in the Jan/Feb 2000 issue of the FDA publication *The Healing Power of Placebos*, "Expectation is a powerful thing. The more you believe you're going to benefit from a treatment, the more likely it is that you will experience a benefit." This is exactly why placebos are used when testing a new drug's medical benefit. If patients on the new drug fare significantly better than those taking a placebo, the study helps support the conclusion that the medicine is responsible for improvements in patients' condition and not the power of positive thinking.

For centuries, unorthodox treatments have produced astounding improvements in health that could not be explained in traditional terms. During the last few decades, researchers have been studying how the placebo effect triggers the mind to regulate and control the body. In 1955, a groundbreaking paper "The Powerful Placebo" demonstrated that 32 percent of patients responded to placebos. Ten years later, breakthrough studies demonstrated that placebos sped up pulse rate, increased blood pressure, and improved reaction speeds when participants were told they had taken a stimulant, but had the opposite effects when participants were told they had taken a sleep-inducing drug.

It's hard for many people to accept the notion that just thinking about curing a disease will often be enough to actually do it; that we can respond as well to an inert pill as we can to an actual drug. But according to Dr. Michael Jospe, a professor at the California School of Professional Psychology, who has studied the placebo effect for more than twenty years, our belief system gives us more healing power than we realize. Jospe points out that all normal people experience physiological reactions to anticipation and stress that help them cope and survive. Each time you experience something and react to it, you learn from it and condition yourself to react before the event even occurs. So the relationship between a thought and a negative reaction is something we experience daily.

That goes for positive associations as well. Also, in the Jan/Feb 2000 issue of the FDA publication *The Healing Power of Placebos,* Dr. Jospe adds, "The placebo effect is part of the human potential to react positively to a healer. You can reduce a patient's distress by doing something that might not be medically effective." He gives the example of children and adhesive bandages. If the adhesive bandage you put on a child's wound has stars or cartoons on it, it can actually make the child feel better by its soothing effect, though there's no medical reason it should make the child feel any better than a plain adhesive bandage. The positive reaction of the child to the images on the bandage seems to make the difference.

In some cases, the placebo may be as good as the actual treatment. One study found that placebos do as well as antidepressants in the majority of patients treated. Other studies have shown that multicolored placebo pills work best overall, green placebos produce better results in anxious or phobic patients, red or orange ones perform better as stimulants, blue ones as sedatives, and yellow ones for depression.[2] Barring some of our new miracle drugs, there are few medications today that have the power of our body's own chemicals.

Amazingly, placebos are also organ-specific. They work exactly the way the actual drug is supposed to work on precisely the body part or organ they're intended to affect. So a placebo taken for joint pain will alleviate the pain in that particular joint, and one taken for a digestive problem will work on the stomach or intestines. One of the best examples of this was illustrated in a Canadian prostate study where more than half the men who had benign enlargement of their prostates were given placebo pills and reported significant relief from their symptoms, including faster urine flow. Researchers theorized that their patients' positive expectations of the drug's benefits caused therapeutic smooth muscle relaxation by decreasing nerve activity to the bladder, prostate, and urethra. In another major placebo study (reported in the Jan/Feb 2000 issue of the FDA publication, *The Healing Power of Placebos),* two-thirds of subjects given a pill they were told would produce severe stomach activity quickly experienced strong stomach churning.

Does the placebo effect work on everyone? No. The answer may lie in individual differences in personality and attitude. Patients who visualize positive outcomes, eliminate stress, and participate in their own healing are the most successful. Those who dwell on the negative and believe that there's no hope experience the "nocebo effect," a negative reaction that depresses the immune system and makes one even more vulnerable to disease. The placebo effect helps prove that having a positive attitude and the will to get better triggers the release of brain chemicals needed for spontaneous healing.

How exactly does the interplay of psychological and physiological mechanisms trigger a healing process that can be as effective as most medicines we take? Today's brain imaging techniques lend support to the theory that thoughts and beliefs not only affect one's psychological state, but also cause the body to undergo actual biological changes. Together, the nervous, endocrine, and immune systems stimulate the release of chemicals that, during emotional responses, sets the healing process in motion.

When you think about it, the human body is an immensely complex system of molecules, which stimulates nerve connections that respond to our mental suggestions. So it makes sense that the placebo effect is really nothing more than a normal immune response. How else can we explain what some people call miracle cures but what more and more doctors refer to as "unexplained spontaneous healing?"

I believe the phenomenon of spontaneous healing occurs because something within us triggers a major response in our immune system, which literally floods our body with increasing white blood cells that attack and destroy whatever is causing the illness. We shouldn't be at all surprised that this happens as often as it does. Without such a response, we'd be dying of diseases at a much more rapid rate. What should surprise us is that we know so little about how to use the mind-body connection to strengthen immunity and spontaneously heal ourselves in the process.

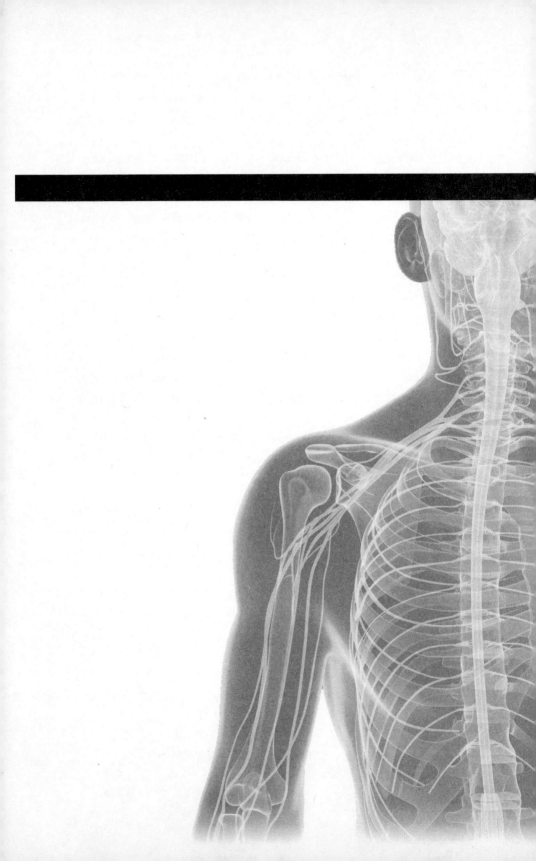

CHAPTER TWO

Why and How We Get Sick

A Mind-Body Perspective

"Mind over matter" is not simply a catchphrase. It is a truth based on what we know to be fact: that the brain, given the right set of directions, the right environment, and the proper stimuli, will always choose healing over disease.

The ability to fend off illness and disease depends on several factors, some of which are beyond your control, but others of which are not. The type of stressor you've been exposed to, such as a pathogen, an injury, or a traumatic event may be—in fact, usually is—beyond your control. But the way you react to the stressor and the general health of your immune system are things you can influence. Harnessing the power of your brain and thus enhancing your ability to boost your immune system is definitely something you can influence. Remember that at the center of it all is the brain, and as we have discussed, the brain is "command central" for the mind and the body.

Homeostasis: An Internal Balancing Act

Each of us has, in our brains, an internal engine that fine-tunes our life processes and keeps us in balance. That engine is homeostasis. For example, when our body temperature increases or decreases too much, homeostatic systems engage to get us back to normal. When our blood sugar gets out of balance, those same systems work to return it to a healthy level. In essence, we stay healthy and disease-free because our body's engine helps keep us within a normal physiological range.

When we lose our ability to get back to that normal range, we set ourselves up for danger. Physical and emotional stress significantly decreases the effectiveness of homeostatic systems by altering biochemical reactions and flooding us with hormones that disrupt life processes. Additionally, as we get older, we don't cope as well with sudden changes because our homeostatic mechanisms aren't as efficient as they once were.

By definition, disease is the failure to maintain homeostasis. Disease is a state of imbalance that usually begins at the tissue level and eventually affects organs or entire organ systems. Sometimes our immune system needs a little help because it doesn't react quickly enough. A bacterial infection, for example, may spread rapidly and overwhelm us unless antibiotics are given to keep the pathogen population down long enough for our own defenses to take over. In most cases, our natural defenses are enough to get the job done, and often we're not even aware that we're being attacked.

A physician friend once told me, "If there was anything in the world I would wish for my patients, it's a healthy and responsive immune system." As long as we have a healthy immune system, the disease process begins and ends fairly quickly. For instance, there is good evidence that cells are making mistakes all the time—including the mistakes that lead to cells becoming cancerous—but the immune system fights back. The body can recognize that a cell is a mutant and destroy it. So we may have cancer for a brief moment of time and then it's gone. Or, we get an infection and our body gets rid of it in short order. It's when our immune system is weakened by internal and external forces that we succumb. A breakdown in homeostasis is often exacerbated by persistent negative thoughts, and the resulting disease may be the product of the mind-body connection working against us.

Neuro-Endocrine-Immune System

One of the most important systems we have to fight disease is really three systems in one. The nervous system, controlled by the brain, regulates the other two: the endocrine and the immune systems. Together, these systems are a veritable army against toxins, pathogens, tissue trauma, and psychological stress, which by itself can cause more disease than the first three factors combined. See Figure 2.1.

Figure 2.1: The Neuro-Endocrine-Immune System

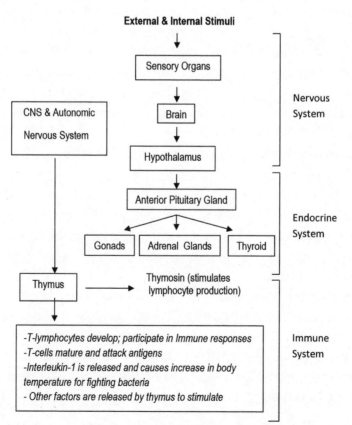

Many diseases besides genetic disorders originate with the nervous system because the brain controls the way all our other organs respond. As discussed earlier, the hypothalamus sends chemical and nerve signals to the pituitary, which in turn releases hormones that trigger chemical reactions and stimulate or inhibit the immune system. In concert, this threesome of organ systems determines how healthy we are and how quickly and effectively we respond to illness when it strikes.

All three of these systems directly affect one another, particularly during embryonic growth and development. And in adulthood the interactions that occur among them depend extensively on a network of chemicals and hormones that travel from one body part to another, sometimes for great distances.

Because the neuro-endocrine-immune system is so interrelated, disruption to one of the organ systems due to a physical challenge like tissue trauma or infection, or a mental challenge that creates stress, typically causes damage to the others. And because this damage usually begins with the brain, our goal should be to ensure that the "neuro" part of the neuro-endocrine-immune system is functioning well. If it isn't, it's that much harder for the body to overcome disease mechanisms.

What Are the Effects of Stress on Health?

If you are not able to change your response to the stressors that are so much a part of modern life, you may find yourself in a continual fight-or-flight reaction. Over time, being effectively stuck in fight-or-flight mode can lead to serious health consequences, including high blood pressure, digestive disorders, or diabetes.

Mind-body therapies and practices can help prevent this. But note that the relationship between stress and illness is not a simple one. There is no simple, direct connection between the number and kinds of stressors you experience, the way you react to those stressors, and how your physical health is affected. But there is a connection.

Some people misinterpret the idea of the mind-body connection and end up blaming themselves for being stressed and sick. This assumes a level of control over their health that isn't realistic. Instead of worrying or self-blaming, do what you can to take care of yourself, including practicing stress management, but it's important to recognize that you don't have complete control.

How Do Mind-Body Therapies Help Reduce Stress?

Mind-body therapies help you change your response to stressors. Some of the ways they can do this include:

- Relaxation response. Many of these therapies invoke the relaxation response. As you may have experienced, the relaxation response reverses the physical effects of stress.

- Positive thinking. Mind-body therapies can also contribute to (or deliberately create) more positive thinking. Evidence shows that people who believe they are doing better actually do better than those who have the same physical condition but aren't as positive. (Research also suggests that anxiety, hostility, depression, and other negative states affect the immune system.)

- Placebo effect. When people believe that a therapy is working, it often does have a positive effect. The placebo effect is often deliberately invoked by mind-body therapies. For example, guided imagery and clinical hypnosis can use suggestions that the patient is getting better.

- Social support is a mind-body therapy in and of itself and is also part of many other mind-body therapies. It has been shown beneficial to health in many studies. "People with supportive social networks have been shown to have better overall health . . . shorter hospital stays when they do get sick, and better resistance to infection than those whose social bonds are not strong."[3]

The principles that make mind-body therapies and practices effective in improving physical health also apply to other aspects of our daily life. These therapies can improve your mental and emotional health and your overall well-being.

Stress and Aging

According to a recent study published in the *Proceedings of the National Academy of Sciences,* there is a direct link between stress and aging. This study compared the chromosomes of thirty-nine women, ages twenty to fifty, who had been caring for children with serious chronic illnesses (and who thus had high levels of stress) with woman caring for healthy children (lower stress).[4]

Women with the highest levels of stress had changes in their chromosomes equivalent to at least one decade of additional aging compared with women with lower stress. But it wasn't only the years of caregiving that related to the change, it was the perception of high stress. Women who had the perception of higher stress levels such as the inability to manage time or feeling overwhelmed by the amount of work, fared the worst. To paraphrase Hans Selye, an Austrian-Canadian endocrinologist and researcher on the responses of organisms to stressors, every stressful experience leaves an indelible scar and exacts a cost—after a stressful situation the organism pays for it by becoming a little older. Given this, could mind-body practices that reduce stress also reduce aging? I'll examine this in a later chapter.

I've included chapters on spirituality, prayer, meditation, and imaging because all of these can have a significant effect on our state of mind and the way we feel and think, which, in turn, can have a profound effect on how our immune system responds to illness and disease.

The Stress Connection

Typically, the main ingredients needed to trigger a disease are an invading foreign substance and a lowered resistance. The invader can be anything from a virus, fungus, parasite, or bacteria to abnormal tissue growth, resulting in a tumor or cancer. The lower the resistance, or the slower the response to the invader is, the more likely the disease will establish itself and overwhelm homeostatic mechanisms. Stress is your body's physiological response to anything you perceive as overwhelming, unpleasant, dangerous, or threatening. In the case of the fight-or-flight response, stress contributes to our survival, enabling us to quickly escape or fight our way out of a threatening situation.

Stress can also be caused by changes we normally think of as positive, such as a job promotion, a new relationship, or the birth of a child. It is excess or ongoing stress that interferes with relationships, work, and social life. Ongoing stress saps your energy resources, causes feelings of negativity and, according to medical research, is responsible for as much as 90 percent of all illnesses and diseases—most notably hypertension, heart disease, and cancer. In addition, stress can be a contributing factor in making existing medical problems worse.

Because each of us is shaped by experiences and a unique genetic makeup, we're all inherently different in how we respond to and deal with stress. At a Biology of Stress conference, Dr. Rachel Yehuda, a research psychologist at Mount Sinai School of Medicine, said, "We don't walk into trauma the same way . . . and we don't walk out of trauma the same way."[5] Yehuda is one of many scientists to show that reactions to stress can vary widely and that outcomes of stressful events arise from a complex interplay between genes and the environment.

Stress makes us all the more susceptible to illness and disease because the brain's hypothalamus sends defense signals to the endocrine system, which then releases an array of hormones that not only get us ready for emergency situations but severely depress immunity as well. Even ordinary, day-to-day activities could push us over the edge, according to David Krantz, PhD of the Uniformed Services University of the Health Sciences, who found that blood flow to the heart is affected by what we're doing and feeling each day and that serious problems can be avoided by keeping track of the simple daily stress in our lives.[6] So just as in other physiological processes, the neuro-endocrine-immune system is at the very heart of the stress response—a series of chemical reactions that affect tissues and organs in ways that can wreak havoc on normal body functions.

It's impossible to say exactly how many different negative reactions occur as a result of physical or emotional stress. What we do know, as indicated in Figure 2.2 below, is that the number is significant.

Figure 2.2: Physical Reactions During the Stress Response

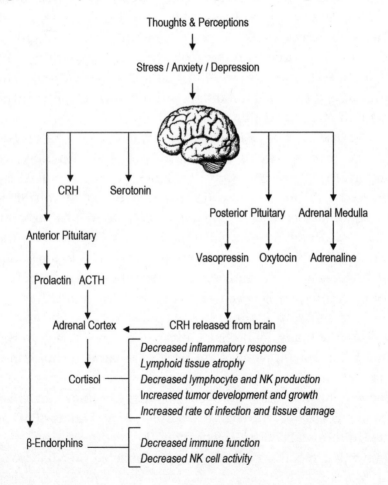

Adapting to Stress

In 1926, a young Hans Selye observed that hospital patients in the early stages of infectious diseases all exhibited similar symptoms, regardless of the type of disease they had. Later, while doing some physiology experiments, he noticed that three common responses occurred whenever any organism was injected with a toxic substance: (1) the adrenal glands enlarged; (2) the lymph nodes and other white-blood-cell producing organs initially swelled and then shrank; and (3) bleeding appeared in the stomach and intestines.

Selye called these three common responses the General Adaptation Syndrome and concluded that certain changes take place within the body during physical stress that disrupt homeostasis and trigger an array of diseases. No matter what type of organism he examined, from rats, dogs, pigs, and monkeys to humans, he found that chronic stress, if left untreated, induced a specific pattern that always led to infection, illness, disease, and eventually death (Figure 2.3). As shown in Hans Selye's General Adaptation Syndrome, various stress reactions occur during each stage that make us more susceptible to disease.

Figure 2.3: Hans Selye's General Adaptation Syndrome

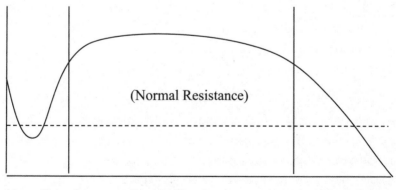

| Alarm Reaction | Stage of Resistance | Exhaustion |

Stage 1: Alarm Reaction: Any physical or mental trauma sets off an immediate set of reactions to combat the stress. Because the immune system is initially depressed, normal resistance levels are lowered, making us more susceptible to infection and disease. If the stress is not severe or long lasting, we bounce back and recover rapidly.

Stage 2: Resistance: Eventually, sometimes rather quickly, we adapt to stress, and there's actually a tendency to become more resistant to illness and disease. Our immune system works overtime for us during this period, trying to keep up with the demands placed upon it. The danger here is that we become complacent and assume that we can resist the effects of stress indefinitely. Believing that we're immune from the effects of stress, we typically fail to do anything about it.

Stage 3: Exhaustion: Because our body is not able to maintain homeostasis, we invariably develop a sudden drop in our resistance level. No one experiences exactly the same resistance and tolerance to stress, but at some point everyone's immunity collapses and is followed by prolonged stress reactions. Life sustaining mechanisms slow down and sputter, organ systems begin to break down, and stress-fighting reserves finally succumb to what Selye called "diseases of adaptation."

While I was a PhD student at Utah State University, my research showed a significant correlation between the emotional stress of oral exams and increased cholesterol and low-density lipoprotein (LDL) levels. Since then other researchers have corroborated my results, showing that total cholesterol and triglycerides can fluctuate by as much as 20 percent during stress and that the bigger the perceived stress the greater the fluctuation in blood lipid levels. LDL, the so-called "bad cholesterol," is especially affected by stress.

The General Adaptation Syndrome is thought to be the main reason why stress is such a prevelant source of health problems. By changing the way our body normally functions, stress disrupts the natural balance—homeostasis—crucial for well-being. It can also subtract years from our lives by speeding up the aging process.

Resistance is the name of the game when it comes to disease. Stress is one of the most significant factors in lowering resistance and triggering the various mechanisms involved in the disease process. By learning the relaxation and stress management techniques found in later chapters, you'll improve your overall health as well as your odds of living a more disease-free life.

Conditioned Immune Responses

Our ancient ancestors evolved what we know as the stress response as a survival mechanism to cope with events in their environment. Similar threats rarely exist in our modern world, thankfully. However, we still respond with the same fight-or-flight stress response—to situations we *perceive* as threatening but may or may not actually be—that, over a lifetime, create an internal environment primed for adverse stress reactions. The longer we allow those events to dominate our thoughts and reactions, the greater the chance they will eventually cause illness and disease.

These conditioned responses increase in strength because they become ingrained into our subconscious and are then triggered by mental or environmental cues. How we perceive events, and the ways in which we react to occurrences in our daily lives, will determine how our brain is conditioned and whether or not we create patterns that contribute more to health or to disease.

One of the more remarkable characteristics of the human brain is how easily it's conditioned. We've all heard about Pavlov's famous dog experiment. Every time Pavlov fed his dog, he would ring a bell. The dog began to associate the sound of the bell with being fed, and eventually, whenever Pavlov rang the bell, the dog would immediately begin salivating. The sound of the bell conditioned the dog's brain to trigger the physiological response of salivating. Humans are no different in that we are just as easily conditioned to sounds, sights, smells, thoughts, and events.

Since the immune system is wired to the brain by a network of blood vessels, and the brain is the major organ of conditioning, immunity and the strength of the immune response depend on two things: (1) how we perceive stimuli and (2) what we do in order to condition ourselves to boost rather than to inhibit immune reactions. Negative perceptions evoke negative reactions, which depress the immune system. The more we evoke negative reactions, the greater the conditioning is and the more such reactions become a spontaneous response (see Figure 2.4).

Figure 2.4: Stress-Induced Conditioning and Habit-Formation

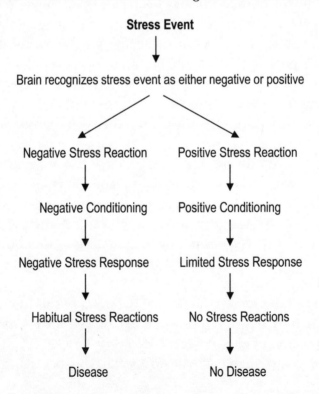

The good news is that we can use fairly simple techniques to create, condition, and reinforce positive responses that help maintain a healthy immune system. There's a lesson to be learned from all this mounting evidence. By strengthening and conditioning the mind part of the mind-body connection in the face of potentially terminal illness, it may be possible to extend life or even recover completely. And by using alternative mind-body techniques in addition to traditional medicine, we'll be doing everything we can to help our body spring into action and do what it needs to do.

Can the Mind Slow Cancer Growth?

Cancer is defined as a group of more than 100 diseases in which abnormal cells divide uncontrollably and then invade other tissues. The term cancer is used to describe not a single disease, but many diseases in which cancer cells begin to grow and then spread to other parts of the body through the blood and lymphatic system. One of the main characteristics of cancer cells is that they're immortal, at least compared to normal cells. The genetic material (DNA) of a cell becomes damaged or changed as a result of chemicals, X-rays, UV rays, or other factors and produces mutations that affect normal cell growth. When this happens, cells don't die when they should and new cells form when the body doesn't need them. The extra cells form a mass of tissue called a tumor.

Treatments for various cancers include chemotherapy, radiation, surgery, or newer procedures like gene therapy and angiogenesis inhibitors. During the past few decades, studies have found that the effectiveness of any of these therapies is enhanced when patients include stress management and other techniques like visualization as part of their overall recovery routine. This is because hormones released during stress reactions not only help cancer cells travel through the bloodstream and spread to other tissues but they help keep those cancerous cells alive and growing by supplying them with vital nutrients. Adding stress management to the mix of cancer treatments may help stimulate the immune system and significantly improve the healing process.

With some exceptions, like breast and colon cancer, few cancers are inherited. Some are the result of defective genes or the environment. The majority, however, are the result of toxins, additives, diets high in saturated fat, industrial and household chemicals, radiation exposure, alcohol, and tobacco. Unfortunately, since the EPA does not test for combinations of chemicals, we really don't know what the effect of exposure to two or more chemicals is on cancer risk compared to single chemical exposure. Research done over the last decade has shown that many people might avoid cancer or would cut their risk significantly if they adhered to seven rules:

1. Don't use tobacco products, including chewing tobacco.

2. Limit sun exposure, especially if you're light-skinned.

3. Avoid food additives and environmental chemicals.

4. Maintain a low-saturated-fat, high-fiber diet.

5. Limit alcohol consumption.

6. Limit sugar intake.

7. Watch your weight.

The one significant risk factor left off the researchers' list is how a person views life events and responds to stress. Human experiments have shown that stress affects key pathogenic processes in cancer such as antiviral defenses, DNA repair, and cellular aging. Conversely, study after study has proven that individuals able to cope with stress are less likely to get cancer. And results from clinical trials have shown that patients who use a variety of stress management techniques and mind-body medicine are much more likely to recover from cancer. Meditation and visualization exercises, for example, improve the general quality of life and can actually enhance the effects of conventional treatment. When chemotherapy or radiation damages white blood cells, along with the cancer cells, the immune system is weakened, which can lead to infection and other diseases. This added stress only fuels the problem and makes stress management and reinforcement of positive thinking even more important.

Beating cancer is never easy. Avoiding the seven risk factors that trigger most cancers is however. Simply following rules number one and five is a way to minimize risk for some of the worst types of cancer such as lung, esophageal, throat, liver, pancreatic, and upper digestive tract. New research has also found that obesity is linked to a dozen types of cancers, including colon, kidney, esophagus, and thyroid, among others. For cancer cells that spring up suddenly without a known cause, maintaining a healthy immune system is the best way to make sure that they are detected, attacked, and eliminated. If researchers have learned anything it's that even a disease like cancer is much more easily overcome when we use the mind-body connection to help fight it. The techniques found throughout the rest of the book will help you do just that.

Are You Cancer-Prone?

More than twenty years ago, an article published by the American Cancer Society asked the question, is there a cancer-prone personality? At the time, results were inconclusive and researchers needed much more information before they could put the debate to rest. Since then, studies have shown that there may indeed be a link between behavior and personality and the onset of and recovery from cancer. We know that emotions such as depression, anger, and hostility make us more prone to illness and disease; and it's been shown that positive attitudes such as hope, optimism, and happiness strengthen our immune system and protect us from disease. Recent studies point to two personality types that seem to make us either cancer-prone or cancer-resistant.[7]

CANCER-PRONE PERSONALITY TYPES

- Represses both positive and negative emotions.

- Shows anger, resentment, or hostility toward others.

- Takes on extra duties and responsibilities, even when they cause stress.

- Reacts adversely to and does not cope well with life changes.

- Is negative or pessimistic.

- Becomes easily depressed or has feelings of hopelessness.

- Has few friends or social networks.

- Worries often and excessively about others.

- Feels the need for approval and to please others.

CANCER-RESISTANT PERSONALITY TYPES

- Expresses emotions in a positive and constructive way.

- Controls anger and resolves anger issues positively.

- Knows when to say no.

- Copes well with stress and feels in control of situations.

- Is optimistic and hopeful.

- Does not become easily depressed.

- Seeks out and maintains social support networks.

- Does not worry excessively.

- Likes to please, but does not seek approval as an emotional crutch.

As with everything else, there are always exceptions: some of the most optimistic and positive among us will get cancer, and some of the angriest and most hostile will live to be 100, cancer-free. Importantly, when a cancer patient is told that his or her disease is terminal, those who adopt cancer-resistant traits tend to live longer because their newly acquired behaviors will automatically boost immunity.

Mind-body techniques such as meditation, autosuggestion, visualization, and relaxation exercises can have a positive effect on cancer treatment. A patient's coping style and recovery strategy are critical factors in five-year survival rates. Mortality is typically reduced for those who have a social support network compared with those who are socially isolated. Patients who establish a recovery program that includes stress management and relaxation techniques have fewer relapses.

A group of researchers at Stanford University found that patients with metastatic breast cancer had a higher quality of life, less pain, and lived at least two years longer if they belonged to a support group, even if they were anxious and depressed about their disease. Their results showed that social support acts as a stress buffer. The patients with cortisol fluctuations had shorter survival times and poorer quality of life, while those who had good family ties and ongoing social support networks had lower cortisol levels and longer survival rates.[8]

There's a lesson to be learned from all this mounting evidence. By strengthening and conditioning the mind part of the mind-body connection, we can extend life and optimize the chances of recovery.

How Stress Affects Cancer Treatment

A common complaint about cancer treatment is "The cure is worse than the disease." Cancer treatments like surgery, chemotherapy, and radiation can be painful and debilitating, both physically and emotionally. The subsequent stress reactions lead to depressed immune function, which then lowers survival rates. A friend of mine who had a rare type of cancer and was undergoing chemotherapy once told me that his treatment was so bad that he felt like just giving up. To him, it seemed as if the treatment was making his disease even worse.

Because cancer treatment can be so stressful in itself and lead to depressed immunity, it's important to keep active and maintain as healthy a lifestyle as possible. Good nutrition is an important part of cancer treatment. Eating the right kinds of foods before, during, and after treatment will go a long way in helping you tolerate the treatment and eventual recovery. According to the American Cancer Society, you need to consume enough nutrients to meet the following goals:

1. Prevent or reverse nutritional deficiencies;

2. Decrease the side effects of the cancer or the treatment; and

3. Maximize the quality of life.

While a healthy diet is always important, it's especially important for people with cancer because it will provide the reserves and strengthen the immune defenses needed to cope with the effects of treatment.

Patients suffering from the physical side effects of chemotherapy and the emotional stress of having cancer will invariably have even lowered immune responses. That's because any kind of stress causes release of cortisol, which blocks the production of natural killer (NK) cells that attack cancer. While recovering from cancer treatment, the last thing a person may want to think about is exercise. But studies have shown that exercise is one of the key factors in improving the quality of life in cancer patients. One study published in 1997 showed that 70 percent of cancer patients experience fatigue during therapy or after surgery and 30 percent of cancer survivors report a loss of energy following treatment, both significant contributors to a decreased quality of life in cancer patients. A subsequent study done in 1998 showed that patients who participated in outpatient wellness programs consisting of aerobic exercise, strength training, flexibility, and relaxation had a 43 percent increase in strength and a 50 percent increase in endurance than those who did not participate.[9]

Both studies linked the benefits of physical activity to a decrease in emotional stress. Many studies since then have corroborated those findings and further concluded that stress management strategies during and after treatment play a vital role in a patient's overall success rate.

Aging and Disease

From the moment we're born we begin to die. Sounds depressing, but the fact is that we begin the aging process at birth and become more susceptible to disease at middle age and especially as we reach sixty years old and beyond. Many diseases normally kept in check by a young, healthy immune system are more likely to overcome a body that can no longer keep up. Chronic diseases disproportionately affect older adults and are associated with disability and diminished quality of life. According to the 2007 US Centers for Disease Control and Prevention (CDC) Report, *CDC's Disaster Planning Goal: Protect Vulnerable Older Adults,* 80 percent of adults over sixty have at least one chronic condition, and 50 percent have at least two.

Some researchers have found that an accumulation of stress over time and age increases the body's production of free radicals. Free radicals are molecules in the body containing unpaired electrons. Damage occurs when the free radical encounters another molecule and seeks to find another electron to pair with its unpaired electron. The free radical often pulls an electron off a neighboring molecule, causing the affected molecule to become a free radical itself. The new free radical can then pull an electron off the next molecule, and a chemical chain reaction of radical production occurs. This process causes damage to cells that contain free radicals. Other research indicates that when older people experience stress they have a lowered lymphocyte count and a decrease in the hormone thymosin, both factors in impaired immune function.

As we age, our homeostatic mechanisms don't work as well as they once did. We don't absorb calcium as well, our digestive and excretory systems are not as efficient, our immune systems are weakened, and our hearts are not as strong. We become less tolerant of stress, both physically and emotionally, which is the reason we don't adjust as well to changes in temperature or blood pressure. We typically recover more slowly from infections, but even more so when we're stressed. According to researchers, HIV-infected patients older than fifty have levels of depression five times higher than the general population, which further increases the risk of other diseases.[10] Not surprisingly, as indicated in Figure 2.5, people are diagnosed with cancer at higher rates as they age.

Figure 2.5: Increase in Cancer Rates as Men and Women Age.

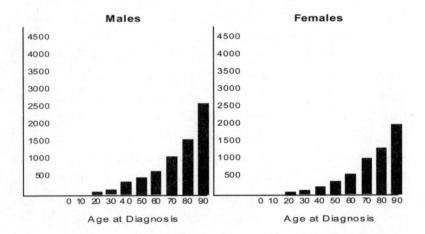

Stress hormones may also contribute to formation of amyloid plaques in the brain and progression of Alzheimer's disease. Researchers at the University of California–Irvine found that when animals were injected with stress hormones, the levels of beta-amyloid production in the brain increased by 60 percent. They also found an increase in the production of another protein called tau, which leads to the formation of tangles, the other signature effect of Alzheimer's. After just one week of experiments, the scientists saw plaque formation in young brains equivalent to brains that were twice as old.

According to Frank LaFerla, PhD, professor of neurobiology and behavior and director of the Institute for Memory Impairments and Neurological Disorders at the University of California–Irvine, managing stress and reducing certain medications that contain glucocorticoids could significantly slow down the progression of Alzheimer's.

Scientists are getting close to discovering the genetic link to aging, which causes cell structure and function to deteriorate. Studies suggest that we are programmed to self-destruct, but that we can postpone that destruction through diet, exercise, and reducing stress. The process of aging itself can trigger various diseases. When a person thinks of aging as a stressful life event, the consequent emotional upheaval will invariably contribute to stress-related illnesses. The more stressful the aging process is perceived to be, the greater the probability that the stress will trigger disease. As a result, it's not unusual to experience some sort of mental health problem as one gets older. Depression is common among the elderly, suicide is higher than it is in any other age group, and phobias and other mental disorders are also high due to four factors:

1. Because the immune system gradually loses its capacity to fight disease, the elderly are more prone to infections and become chronically sick. This leads to preoccupation with mortality and the onset of emotional disorders. Depression and suicide increase when physical and mental activities decrease.

2. Sensory and motor functions decline, which frustrate most older individuals. They are less likely to initiate a daily exercise program or to maintain healthful lifestyles because they feel as if nothing they do will help.

3. Continued stress reactions lead to negative conditioning. This habitual reinforcement strengthens the stress response and causes even more illness and disease.

4. The elderly typically have decreased social interactions. This is especially true after a spouse dies, following an illness, or when children move away. Rather than getting involved in activities that enhance their social support, they become isolated and depressed.

Despite the fact that we succumb to more diseases as we age, life expectancy has been rising steadily. Worldwide, the average lifespan is expected to extend another ten years by 2050. In the United States, the numbers of adults over the age of sixty-five will more than double by 2030, as will the number of adults over the age of eighty. The reasons are improved nutrition, more activity, decreased rates of smoking, and better health practices such as stress management that keep our immune systems working better and longer.

No matter what we might wish, no one has as yet discovered the elusive Fountain of Youth, and we are nowhere near a breakthrough that will reverse aging or stop the programmed end of life. What we can do is make sure that life ends naturally and not with a disease that could have been avoided. In the chapters ahead, I'll discuss ways in which we can condition the brain to help us slow the aging process and maximize life span. I'll also discuss proven methods for boosting the immune system and fighting disease throughout life, no matter how old we are.

CHAPTER THREE

Using the Mind-Body Connection to Prevent Disease

Recognizing Signs and Symptoms

Reversing the disease process and maintaining health and well-being throughout life is not as challenging as it sounds, so long as we maintain a regular program of prevention and, when necessary, intervention. Regular checkups, screenings (blood pressure, cholesterol, prostate and mammary exams, etc.), healthy diet, exercise, stress management, and even alternative treatments are all part of a strategy that keeps our immune system strong and healthy.

A *sign* is the physical effect caused by a particular disease: an unusual lump, a lesion, a change in skin color. A *symptom* is what we feel to be a change in our normal bodily function: pain, nausea, fatigue, etc. Some diseases affect very limited body areas. Carcinogens, for example, affect only certain cells in certain parts of the body. Therefore, we need to be aware of any changes and not ignore symptoms, even if we don't think they're very serious. Keep in mind, though, that we all have different levels of tolerance. A small irritant to one person can actually be a major symptom that indicates the beginnings of a disease.

Under no circumstance should we try to diagnose ourselves. That's what people spend years in medical school and residency programs for. But what we can do is look for early warning signs and symptoms that, once discovered, should always be discussed with our physician or healthcare provider. It's easy to overlook small, insignificant things or to chalk symptoms up to nothing more than minor aches or pains. And though we don't want to become hypochondriacs, misdiagnosis is a common way to allow a disease that could have been treated at an early stage to progress and get out of hand, in some cases becoming incurable.

By looking and feeling for changes regularly, you'll be more aware of them when they do eventually happen. Some of us may not like the idea of inspecting ourselves; we may feel its immodest or just "not how we were raised." But how else do we become familiar enough with our body to know what it normally should look and feel like?

Symptoms are divided into how they affect us physically, mentally, emotionally, and behaviorally. And though many common signs and signals of stress reactions can mimic symptoms of other problems, or do not lead to serious disease, they certainly might. The following table lists the most common signs to look for in the physical, mental, and emotional spheres, as well as the behavioral signs.

Common Signs and Signals of a Stress Reaction

Physical	Mental	Emotional	Behavioral
Fatigue	Blaming others	Anxiety	Changes in normal activities
Insomnia	Confusion	Guilt/ Self-Blame	Change in speech
Muscle tremors	Poor attention	Grief	Withdrawal
Twitching	Unable to make decisions	Denial	Emotional outbursts
Difficulty breathing	Heightened or lowered alertness	Moodiness	Change in communication in amount or content, becoming quiet or too verbal, or abrupt/hostile in tone
Rapid breathing	Poor concentration	Fear of Loss	
Hypertension	Forgetfulness	Uncertainty	
Rapid heartbeat	Trouble identifying known objects or people	Loss of emotional control	
Chest pain		Emotional numbness	Suspiciousness
Headaches	Decreased awareness of surroundings	Depression	Inability to rest
Visual difficulties		Lack of capacity for enjoyment	Substance abuse
Nausea/ Vomiting	Poor problem-solving	Apprehension	Intensified startle reflex
Excessive thirst	Loss of sense of time, place, or person	Intense anger	Antisocial acts
Hunger		Irritability	Pacing
Dizziness	Disturbed thinking	Agitation	Erratic movements
Excess sweating	Nightmares	Helplessness	Decreased hygiene
Chills	Inescapable images	Mistrust	Diminished sex drive
Weakness		Feelings of worthlessness	Appetite disturbance
Fainting	Flashbacks	Apathy/ Boredom	Prolonged silences
Diarrhea	Suicidal ideas	Irritability	Accident prone
Stomach pains	Disbelief	Disorientation	Teeth grinding
	Change in values		Increased smoking
	Search for meaning		Foot tapping
	Feelings of panic		Nervous laughter
	Nightmares		

These symptoms don't necessarily indicate disease. But stress always leaves an unmistakable pattern of signs and symptoms, followed by stress-related illnesses. Not heeding our body's signals can be a serious mistake because diseases frequently manifest themselves early on as dull aches, sharp pains, nervous twitches, nausea, numbness, or sudden throbbing in a particular area of the body.

We must also keep in mind that pain isn't always the first sign of a disease process. In cancer, for example, there is usually no pain at all until the disease progresses and begins to affect nerve cells and destroy the sensitive tissue surrounding the tumor. The American Cancer Institute lists the seven early warning signs of cancer so that the first letter of each sentence spells the word "caution."

- **C**hange in bowel function or bladder control and/or habits.

- **A** sore that persists, spreads, or does not heal.

- **U**nusual bleeding or discharge.

- **T**hickness or a lump in tissue such as the breast, testis, etc.

- **I**ndigestion or difficulty in swallowing.

- **O**bvious change in the shape of a mole, wart, or blemish.

- **N**agging cough or a persistent sore throat.

Recognizing early warning signs is critical in treatment success rates and significantly improves recovery. Prostate cancer, one of the leading causes of cancer deaths in men, is one of the most curable cancers when caught early. Tragically, men don't discuss prostate cancer with other men or their sons, they fail to get regular prostate screenings like they should, and they are not diagnosed early enough to get effective treatment.

Personality also plays a role in how we recognize symptoms and how intensely we feel those symptoms when we get them.

An individual with a Type A personality, for example, may assume that his or her symptoms are nothing more than the unpleasant consequence of work. He or she will become more tolerant of sudden changes or ignore them altogether. It may be one of the reasons Type A individuals have more heart attacks and develop hypertension and other diseases.

The bottom line in recognizing signs and symptoms is to pay attention to even small, seemingly insignificant signals that indicate any change from normal. Homeostatic systems are very sensitive. When our body gets away from normal, it tells us something is wrong; and that's exactly why learning to listen to our body is so important in preventing diseases from getting out of hand. The first step in treating stress is to notice the signs and signals. Sometimes just knowing that our body is telling us we're stressed is enough to help us overcome it.

Stress Intervention as Preventive Medicine

When left unchecked, stress is a principal contributing factor in virtually every human disease. Managing stress can be relatively simple. Pinpointing the source of that stress in order to prevent disease may not be as easy. So how do we determine what's causing our stress? One surefire way is by knowing our body and linking signs and symptoms to stress sources through the use of a stress diary.

For years I've been teaching people how to identify hidden sources of stress. The reason my method has been successful is because it's simple, easy to use, and effective. Within three weeks, individuals keeping a stress diary uncover sources of stress that are often difficult to identify because they've been incorporated into daily life and are no longer obvious or unique. Hidden sources of stress are the most dangerous because they are left alone to trigger stress reactions and cause continued wear and tear on the body's immune system.

Here's an example of a stress diary from one of my stress management seminars. It's not necessary to have one exactly like this, but since this type has worked so well in the past, I suggest starting out by using this one as your model.

Day / Date _____

Time of Day	Stress Symptom	Immediate Activity	Previous Activity
8:00 a.m.	Headache	Cooking breakfast	Making school lunches
12:00 p.m.	Neck pain	Eating lunch	Paying bills
4:00 p.m.	Biting fingernails	Doctor's visit	Thinking about unpaid bills
10:00 p.m.	Stomach pains	Watching TV	Arguing with son
12:00 p.m.	Insomnia	Reading in bed	Anger about argument

Because even the most negative stressors can become incorporated as routine events, or habits, into our lives, the only way to eliminate them is to keep an accurate record of activities, emotions, and thoughts that invariably lead to the symptoms they produce. As soon as you notice a symptom, write it down, along with the time of day or night it occurred, the type of activity you were doing at the time, as well as any thoughts or activities prior to that one. It's important to include thoughts as well as physical activities, since thoughts can be even more potent triggers of stress reactions than actual events.

Just as important as immediate events are any prior/ proximate thoughts and activities because stress reactions don't always occur at the same time we encounter stressors that cause those reactions. In many cases, symptoms may not be evident right away. They can manifest themselves hours later. Therefore, to get a true indication of what may really be causing symptoms, look back and remember what you were experiencing during the past few hours.

Regardless of how insignificant you might think your thoughts and actions seem, write them down. What might appear insignificant at the time could turn out to be the major cause for triggering the symptoms you're experiencing. After a week of keeping a stress diary, you can begin to look for patterns. When I'm working with individuals, I have them ask themselves three sets of questions.

1. Are symptoms more noticeable during certain times? Do the symptoms disappear when I alter the time that I do specific activities? Is nighttime better? Does reorganizing my schedule make what I'm doing produce less symptoms?

2. Is what I'm doing causing the symptoms? Am I too intense in doing what I'm doing? Do I worry the entire time? Do I use so much energy that I feel worn out as a result? Is it really necessary to do the activity in the first place? Can I do without it? When I stop, do the symptoms go away?

3. Is how I'm acting when doing the activity causing symptoms? Is the amount of time spent doing the activity causing symptoms? Do I spend too much time or too little? Is the amount of time spent on the activity keeping me from doing other more important things?

The answers to these questions give you a pretty good idea of what's causing your symptoms and why the things you do or the feelings you have make you sick. Keeping a diary is a great way to catch small things early on and prevent them from becoming the big things that disrupt homeostatic mechanisms, depress the immune system, and trigger disease.

Keeping a diary, however, means you have to follow through and do something about your stress symptoms. So at the end of the diary period, write down three important facts: (1) the cause of your symptoms, (2) the reason for your symptoms, and (3) the solution to your problem. Here's an example using headaches as the stress symptom:

Cause of symptom: rushing to make lunches for the kids each morning; feeling as if everyone is going in opposite directions.

Reason(s) for symptom: feeling as if not enough time to do everything that's needed—to sit, talk, and have breakfast together.

Solution:

1. Set the alarm for thirty minutes earlier.

2. Prepare lunches and clothing the night before.

3. Get better organized in the mornings; don't leave things to be done till the last minute.

The better we get at recognizing the things that are causing symptoms, the easier it will be to intervene and come up with solutions to eliminate the source of the problem. Sometimes just recognizing that our symptoms are being caused by simple, day-to-day activities brings considerable relief and we immediately begin to feel better and healthier. In many cases, the simple act of discovering why we are having symptoms makes us more aware of ways we can solve the problem.

Another good use for a symptom diary is to track how well supplements and medications are working. If you want to try an herbal product instead of Prozac to combat depression, for example, keep a record of exactly when and where you get depressed and whether taking the herbs alleviates some of those symptoms. The diary will also tell you what, if anything, is likely triggering your depression in the first place. In later chapters, I'll discuss proven methods and solutions for eliminating non-clinical depression and anxiety and the stress that often leads to symptoms and eventually to diseases related to it.

How Sleep Affects the Mind-Body Connection

We've all experienced what it's like to go without enough

sleep. We become irritable, moody, and mentally fatigued. Our sex lives suffer. And we become more susceptible to colds, infections, and more serious illnesses and disease. Sleep is critical for the proper function of the neuro-endocrine-immune system, which works to maintain both physical and mental well-being.

Researchers are finding that even something as simple as a power nap enhances information processing and learning. Experiments by scientists at the National Institute of Mental Health and Harvard University show that a midday snooze reverses information overload and can improve learning a motor skill by 20 percent.[11] Their studies suggest that during sleep, the brain consolidates the memories of habits, actions, and skills learned during the day. So rather than feeling guilty about catching a few extra winks, we should use them to rejuvenate.

During the past few decades, sleep researchers have shown sleep to be a powerful mechanism that boosts immune function and restores the body's homeostatic mechanisms. Some of our hormones are elevated, others decreased; tissues are repaired more rapidly; and we gradually bring ourselves back to a state of normal equilibrium. In essence, we give ourselves a chance to regenerate and recuperate from some of the bad or stressful things we've done to ourselves.

Electroencephalogram (EEG) studies have shown that brain activity during sleep is either present as normal brain waves or is being disrupted throughout the night. A normal eight-hour sleep pattern consists of five main stages of sleep, each characterized by different brain waves. Periods of rapid eye movement known as REM sleep are interspersed with quieter periods called non-REM sleep stages. About 25 percent of the night is spent in REM, and someone who spends eight hours sleeping will typically go through all five stages four or five times. The stages are:

Stage I: Fleeting thoughts enter one's mind but the brain waves become smaller. This is sometimes called "dozing," in which breathing is slower and more regular, the mind wanders, and pulse rate decreases. Stage I only lasts for a few minutes.

Stage II: Brain waves become larger and slower during this period, which lasts about fifteen to twenty minutes. There are sudden bursts of electrical activity. Eyes do not move and are not responsive. There is very little muscular activity.

Stage III: Brain waves slow significantly but are larger than in stage II. This stage is sometimes known as "Slow Wave Sleep." Sleep here is deep and restful and lasts about 30 minutes. The body is very relaxed, breathing slows, and heart rate decreases.

Stage IV: As one reaches this final stage of non-REM sleep, there is deep relaxation. In fact, muscles are so relaxed that the body is essentially paralyzed. However, pulse and breathing rate quickens and blood flow increases.

REM: Brain waves speed up to the same pattern seen when the person is awake. It is during this period that one experiences the greatest amount of dreaming. Lasting anywhere from a few minutes to almost an hour, the total muscle relaxation during REM normally prevents one from acting out the dream.

The latest research suggests that for adults seven hours is the minimum amount of sleep needed to keep the mind-body connection working at its best. Studies have found that people who sleep an average of eight hours a night live longer than people who don't sleep as well; and those suffering from sleep disorders like insomnia, or who have disrupted sleep patterns, are at greater risk for chronic illness. Shift workers, for example, sleep less on average than non-shift workers and, because their sleep patterns are fragmented, are never able to recover from the day's work.

Although we don't sleep as much at fifty as we did at twenty, it's not true that we require less sleep as we get older. Sleep patterns need to be consistent for us to maintain good health. But it's not always easy to maintain good sleep habits as we age because our minds and our bodies change. Older individuals don't make brain chemicals in the same amounts as do younger individuals, and the brain doesn't respond to those chemicals as effectively. As we age, we also have more things on our minds, we get stressed out by more complex issues, we become depressed more often and, as a result, the quality of our sleep suffers.

Inability to sleep may be a symptom of a more serious physical or emotional problem. So if the suggestions in this section don't work for you, you probably need to consult a physician to determine if there's a more serious underlying issue. Disrupted sleep patterns are often caused by physical ailments, chemical imbalances, or mental health problems such as depression. The three main categories of sleep disorders are:

Parasomnia: These are abnormal behaviors during sleep like talking, walking, grinding teeth, etc. In these cases, the skeletal muscles are not fully relaxed. The problem is usually physical, but there may be some underlying psychological problem involved as well.

Insomnia: This is inability to fall asleep or having shortened sleep periods. As many as 30 percent of adults have this common sleep disorder, which is caused by a variety of factors such as stress, depression, drug use, lifestyle, or poor nighttime habits.

Hypersomnia: The opposite of insomnia, hypersomnia is excessive sleep. An individual may sleep for more than twelve hours and also take naps. The cause may be either physiological or psychological. Depression, for example, may cause a person to want to escape from reality or to avoid situations by sleeping as much as possible.

Maintaining good health doesn't only include nutrition and exercise. Normal sleep patterns are critical for both physical and mental health. The worst thing you can do is sleep a full eight hours one night and then six another, or go to bed at ten o'clock on Monday night and after midnight on Tuesday. All you're doing is continually resetting your biological clock and falling into a pattern of insomnia. The best way to get back on track is not by taking sleeping pills but by changing your sleep-related habits and behaviors. Here are some of the suggestions that have helped people break their disruptive nighttime habits and get back into a healthy sleep pattern. Within weeks, you'll not only feel more energized but you'll be reversing the wear and tear your body has gone through because of poor sleep.

- **Maintain a regular sleep schedule.**
  We all have a finely tuned biological clock that helps us sleep and wake up. Whenever we disrupt that clock by continually changing it, we set ourselves up for sleepless nights and chronic fatigue. It then takes a while for our brain to readjust and reset. To avoid creeping insomnia, develop a routine so that your body knows when it's time to transition from being awake to sleep.

- **Don't try to catch up too much on weekends.**
  Many of us do it: stay up late on Friday and Saturday and sleep in too late on Saturday and Sunday morning. The problem with that is that our internal clock readjusts itself by Sunday evening and we're back to tossing and turning when we go to bed. So even if you stay up late on weekends, force yourself to get up not more than an hour later than you normally do.

- **Avoid caffeine at night, especially before bed.**
  Coffee and energy drinks are big culprits, but be aware of other products that contain caffeine as well. Soft drinks, chocolate, and certain medications may contain just enough to keep you awake, especially if you consume too

much of them. A good rule of thumb is to avoid caffeine at least four hours before bed.

- **Don't get over stimulated before bedtime.**
Using your mind and thinking too much right before bed will often stimulate rather than tire you out. The brain needs to know when it's time for sleep, and clearing the mind of distractions helps maintain that sensitive internal biological clock. If you find that watching TV or reading a thriller before bed keeps you up, change your habits by relaxing and reading something less exciting.

- **Drink warm milk before bed.**
Milk contains tryptophan, an amino acid that's converted to serotonin, which induces sleep. If you're hungry, you might want to add some protein powder to the milk. Avoid simple carbohydrates, as these spike your insulin levels and disrupt normal sleep patterns.

- **Avoid alcohol at night.**
Because alcohol is a central nervous system depressant, a few drinks can make you sleepy. However, while alcohol initially causes you to become tired, sleep will not last more than a few hours because alcohol disrupts normal sleep cycles. Furthermore, people who depend on a drink every evening condition themselves to become dependent on alcohol in order to fall asleep.

- **Don't exercise late in the evening.**
Exercise not only increases heart rate, blood pressure, and blood flow to the brain, it also triggers a surge of other hormones that flood the body and keep us stimulated for hours. To avoid this, the best time to exercise is morning or late afternoon.

- **Avoid drinking too much water immediately before bed.**
A glass or two of water right before bed will wake you up a few hours later to go to the bathroom. If you have

trouble going back to sleep once you're awake, this is not a habit you want to get into. If it happens on a regular basis, the "routine" becomes so conditioned that your internal clock will begin to wake you up at a certain time each night, whether you need to "go" or not.

- **Sleep on a good quality, comfortable mattress.**
Something as simple as changing your mattress can prevent aches and pains that disrupt sleep. Most people are helped by a firmer mattress that doesn't create swells that cause bends in the body. Some of the newer memory foam mattresses that conform to your body curves are excellent.

- **Keep your bedroom cool and dark.**
The optimum temperature for sleep is sixty-eight degrees because that's the temperature that seems to best set the brain's internal thermostat. The mild drop in body temperature induces sleep. Blocking out all light triggers the pineal gland to produce melatonin, the hormone that tells your body it's time to sleep. A night light, and even a light on the alarm clock next to your bed, will confuse the pineal and disrupt sleep.

- **Take magnesium an hour before bed.**
If your sleep is disrupted by anxiety, or if you're tossing and turning because you're thinking about things that cause you stress, magnesium may be the answer. This supplement has a calming effect on the nerves and helps relax muscles so that you sleep more soundly. Because sleep deprivation is stressful, and since stress lowers magnesium levels, taking a magnesium supplement may help get you back in balance.

- **Stretch before going to bed.**
Tension and muscle pain can keep you from getting to sleep or can wake you up in the middle of the night. Ten minutes of yoga or stretching will relieve the tension and help you stay more relaxed throughout the night.

• **Avoid foods that cause insomnia.**
If you're having trouble dozing off, what you eat before bed may be sabotaging your sleep. Foods to avoid are: deli meats like ham, sausage, pepperoni, bacon, and smoked meats because they contain tyramine, which triggers the release of brain stimulants and makes you restless; spicy foods because they raise body temperature and may cause heartburn; and high-fat meals because they can disrupt natural sleep cycles.

• **Relax with some stress management exercises.**
Relaxation exercises and meditation have natural tranquilizing effects that induce sleep. By practicing these before bed, you'll be conditioning the brain to trigger a deeply relaxed state that can easily transition your body into sleep.

We don't realize how important sleep is until we start having sleep problems that leave us tired, irritable, and unproductive. Because the physical effects of sleep deprivation are cumulative, they lead to lowered disease resistance. Adapting good sleep habits will not only make us feel more refreshed and energized but will keep us a lot healthier as well.

How We Think Really Matters

The way we perceive daily events, the way we view the world around us, the manner in which we respond to stress and interact with others all affect the way in which our body maintains homeostasis. The reason it's called the mind-body connection is because the mind is working in sync with the body to process the multitude of reactions that control every organ system. We think and then we respond. And how we respond is basically a matter of mind over body.

Simply put, life events are viewed as either good or bad depending on how we choose to look at them. One of my students actually enjoyed getting into traffic jams because it gave him an opportunity to think and reflect on things in his life. While many of us would be ready to explode into a rage at being stuck on a highway and going nowhere, he would use the time to do something constructive like listening to the radio and catching up on current news events or mentally reviewing facts for an upcoming exam. It's attitude more than anything else. And attitudes, just like habits, are conditioned responses that can be changed for the better. If you're thinking that this is easier said than done, consider how quickly we can form habits or how easily we condition ourselves to behave in certain ways. With a little effort, we can just as easily condition ourselves to develop attitudes that bring out the best in us.

Okay, so you accept that you have a bad attitude; and you'd really like to feel and think differently. But exactly how do you change attitudes in order to prevent illness and disease? The answer is not to try to change your personality but to make small adjustments in your outlook and behavior that, over time, will automatically change the attitudes that are affecting health. Sometimes the best and most effective preventive medicine is conditioning the brain to perceive life events in a new way. Here are eleven suggestions I offer in my seminars that people have found help them the most.

- **View change as rewarding and challenging.** In most cases, change is not something we view positively. Many of us are not very good at it; and the older we get the harder it becomes. Sometimes it's simply a fear of the unknown or the fear of failure. So rather than viewing change as something negative, look for the positives. The more consistently we do that, the less negatively we'll feel about change in general.

- **Visualize positive results.** As if we're looking through someone else's eyes, we visualize what's happening to us or what will happen to us, and we don't like what we see. Performance anxiety is common when we're about to give a speech or have sex or perform some other function. To rid yourself of this negative habit, imagine success instead of failure. Once you condition the brain to see positive outcomes, you'll overcome that initial urge to think the worst.

- **Take control over situations.** Having a feeling of control is one of the most important and fundamental attitudes we can have to combat stress and prevent illness. Studies have shown that we get sick, not as a result of stressful situations, long hours, job pressures, or low pay but rather from feelings that what we do is beyond our control. The best way to reverse that is to get involved rather than to sit passively by and have others take charge. Join, participate, volunteer, and become active. Doing whatever you can to lead instead of follow will make you feel more in control, even if you're not.

- **Don't be a perfectionist.** Since perfection does not exist, trying to be perfect can lead to burnout, isolation, depression, and eventually disease. It's okay to try and be the best we can be. But what we need to come to grips with is the fact that there will be always be things we can't do as well as we'd like. We have to accept that and move on.

- **Discover your peak energy levels.** Each of us has a unique internal biological clock. Some of us are morning people; others have more energy during the afternoon or evening. By discovering what type of person we are, we can avoid stressful or strenuous situations that sap our energy levels and make us feel as if we're not accomplishing what we should. On the other hand, scheduling the most difficult tasks around peak energy times makes us more efficient. Recognizing when we're at our best is a good first step in eliminating burnout, limiting wear and tear on the body, and keeping our immune system healthy and functioning well.

- **Take time out.** Everyone—no matter how much they love what they're doing or how stress-tolerant they think they may be—needs time to help their homeostatic mechanisms recover from the work they've done. At work, we need to take a few minutes every two hours or so to relax and get ourselves back into a good frame of mind. We should never skip lunch if we don't have to, and we should try to do something special on occasion to make ourselves feel important.

- **Stress-proof your surroundings as much as possible.** Our environment and the things that surround us can have a profound impact on how we feel and how energized we are. If we listen to music, we need to listen only to the type of music that makes us feel relaxed, not the music that's currently popular or that we think we should be listening to. Surround yourself and decorate your home and office with pictures you enjoy looking at and with color schemes that are soothing rather than stimulating.

- **Don't dwell on the past.** It's important not to get caught up in past events. Dwelling too much on previous failures, on what we should have done or said, conditions the brain to intensify those negative thoughts the next time. The past is over, and the only thing we can do is work on the present and prepare for the future. Instead of worrying about what should have been, our past experiences can be used as a tool for focusing on future accomplishments. The most accomplished people in life, the most successful entrepreneurs, the greatest scientists and achievers all have one thing in common: they all learn from past mistakes and they all use failure as an incentive to accomplish what they set out to do.

- **Begin an exercise program.** There's more to exercise than simply getting fit. Regular exercise boosts our immune system and makes us fight disease more effectively. It energizes us, helps us relax, improves sex life, increases resistance, and gives us an overall feeling of health and well-being. Stimulating the body refreshes the mind. Our brain requires activity by the rest of the body in order to revitalize the senses and keep us in a constant state of balance. Individuals who exercise at least three times a week are significantly more likely to trigger the strong immune responses needed to combat disease.

- **Express your feelings.** The simple act of expressing ourselves has a dramatic effect on how we feel and cope with life events. Psychologists working with people who have post-traumatic stress disorder (PTSD) find that patients recover more quickly and are sick less often the more they become comfortable talking about the event that caused the trauma. Studies done since the 1980s have shown that writing about an experience dulls its emotional impact, helps lead to successful recovery, and actually produces stronger immune responses. This "journal therapy" technique can have a profound effect on our health by interfering with disease processes.

- **Learn to say no.** If you are always a "yes" person, you're less likely to feel in control and more likely to get sick. The reason is simple. Those who can't say no often get overextended, usually feel like they're being taken advantage of, and are angered at their helplessness and passive behavior. As a result, they become stressed out and never seem to find time for what they want to do for themselves. Delaying a decision is a good technique to use because it allows us to remove ourselves from the situation and gives us time to find an excuse. We can simply respond with, "Let me check my schedule and get back with you." Then we can decide if we want to get involved or we can come up with some legitimate excuse we were unable to think of on the spur of the moment.

A few simple changes in how we live our day-to-day lives can have a significant effect on our ability to prevent illness and disease. Using even some of these suggestions will go a long way to conditioning our brain to elicit strong and healthy immune responses.

Nutrition and Disease Prevention

Do nutritional supplements like vitamins, minerals, and herbs prevent disease? The jury is still out, and research is ongoing, but in general, yes. In many cases, supplements are intended to replenish nutrients lost during normal activities and especially during stress. Sometimes the only reason we feel tired and fatigued is because we need that infusion of vitamins and minerals, which keep our organs functioning properly. Whenever we feel good physically, we have a better outlook on life, which then translates into a healthy mind and a healthy immune system.

Vitamins are organic compounds required in tiny amounts to maintain bodily functions and fuel chemical reactions. Minerals are naturally occurring substances that are critical in physiological mechanisms such as nerve conduction, bone growth, blood formation, muscle contraction, and heart rate. When the body is stressed or it needs to fight off disease or infection, it actually needs more minerals than vitamins. The foods we eat are usually the best sources of vitamins and minerals. Unfortunately, we don't always eat the right foods, and the stress we're under may require more nutrients than we're getting. So it's often smart to supplement our diet with vitamins and minerals, as long as we're aware of potential side effects.

Studies have shown the benefits of nutritional supplements in disease prevention, especially during aging. One reason is that free radicals, which cause wear and tear on organ systems, are reduced by certain vitamins like C and E. Vitamins have also been shown to strengthen the immune system in general, which then translates into a healthier body and a positive attitude. A positive attitude, in turn, keeps the immune system humming. Here are the vitamins most critical in maintaining essential life processes and the foods they are found in:

Vitamin A: cantaloupes, carrots, broccoli, dark green leafy vegetables, red and green peppers, spinach, sweet potatoes, tomatoes, liver, dairy products, and fish.

Vitamin B6: bananas, peas, turnip greens, carrots, sweet potatoes, chicken, eggs, liver, and fish.

Vitamin B12: liver, milk, eggs, cheese, crab, tuna, lamb, veal, poultry, and fish.

Vitamin C: broccoli, green peppers, potatoes, tomatoes, grapes, grapefruit, and oranges.

Vitamin D: beef, chicken, egg yolk, liver, fortified milk, salmon, tuna, and other fatty fish.

Vitamin E: sweet potatoes, whole wheat bread, shrimp, peanuts, pecans, sunflower seeds, and almonds.

Vitamin K: asparagus, broccoli, Brussels sprouts, cabbage, green leafy vegetables, ham, lettuce, liver, pistachios, spinach, Swiss chard, vegetable oils, turnip greens.

The FDA has found that most dietary supplements are safe when used properly. There are a few herbal products, however, that have been classified as unsafe by the FDA and the US Department of Agriculture (USDA). Some have been issued warnings that they may interfere with other medications; others are extremely toxic and are known to cause cancer. The following chart, according to health agencies, includes the biggest culprits.

Herb	Possible Side Effects
Aristolochia	Kidney failure and cancer of the urinary tract
Ashwagandha	Increases muscle contractions and may induce abortions
Borage Seed	Stomach disorders and/or liver damage
Calamus	Dizziness, nausea, and hallucinations
Cat's Claw	Diarrhea and hypotension; patients with lupus may experience kidney failure.
Chaparral	Commonly called the creosote bush and sold as a cancer treatment, it may cause irreversible liver failure.
Coltsfoot	Tumors and liver cancer
Comfrey	Originally used to reduce swelling, it may cause cirrhosis and eventual liver failure.
Echinacea	Upset stomach, diarrhea, constipation, skin rashes, and dizziness
Ephedra	Also called ma huang, it has been linked to at least 100 deaths due to cardiac arrest and stroke.
Eucalyptus	Dermatological problems, convulsions, and seizures
Fenugreek	Diarrhea, GI bleeding, and hypoglycemia
Foxglove	Nausea, vomiting, and in some cases cardiac arrest; also interacts adversely with prescription drugs.
Germander	A common name for a group of plants that are contained in medicinal tea, it may cause hepatitis, breathing problems, and chest pain.
Kava	Fatigue, liver damage
Lobelia	Known as Indian tobacco, it may cause nausea and vomiting; also interferes with other medications.
Pennyroyal	Nerve damage, convulsions, and seizures
Pokeweed	Nausea, vomiting, diarrhea, and rapid heart rate
Ragwort	Liver damage and breathing problems
Sassafras	Hallucinations, high blood pressure, increased heart rate, muscle spasms, paralysis, and liver cancer
Senna	Stomach cramps, diarrhea, and heart arrhythmia

Herb	Possible Side Effects
St. John's Wort	Used to treat mild depression, it may interact with other medications like protease inhibitors and lessen their effectiveness; it may also cause dizziness, headaches, confusion, and GI disturbances.
Willow Bark	Used for pain and inflammation, it may cause stomach burning, nausea, bleeding ulcers, and liver damage.
Yohimbe	A tree bark that may cause renal failure, seizures, anxiety, panic attacks, stomach disorders, paralysis, and cardiac arrest.

Diets That Fight Disease

Just as surely as certain foods—those high in saturated fat, for example—can make us more susceptible to disease, many foods can make us feel more energized and mentally alert, and can keep us healthy by maintaining the neuro-endocrine-immune system in top working order. Some foods—those rich in fiber and those that are not processed—actually cleanse the digestive system, ridding the body of synthetics and toxins that would otherwise end up in the bloodstream and contaminate the body.

An added benefit to eating foods that revitalize us and make us feel better is the psychological effect these feelings have on us. Simply feeling better strengthens immunity and thus helps prevent disease. On a subconscious level, we get the message that feeling good means being healthy. I've described how vitamins and minerals can help us fight off illness and disease. Here are a few health and nutritional tips that boost energy levels, maintain the immune system, and keep the mind-body connection working at full capacity.

- **Eat well-balanced meals.** Most of us aren't as conscientious as we should be about getting all the daily nutrients we need. Supplements aren't a perfect substitute, but they do offer us a way to ensure that we at least get what we need to stay healthy.

- **Never skip breakfast.** Breakfast eaters are less likely to be obese and more likely to have good blood sugar levels and lower cholesterol. They also stay full longer and have more energy throughout the day. Skip the doughnuts and sugary cereals, however, and choose something healthy like oatmeal, eggs, yogurt, or whole grains.

- **Approach with caution: low-calorie diets.** When your car is running out of gas, you stop to refill it. It's no different with your body, which uses the calories from food to supply energy and power your muscles. How many calories you need each day depends on your age, weight, gender, and how active you are. Starving yourself will not only make you feel sluggish and irritable, it also lowers your metabolism and makes it harder for you to maintain proper weight in the long run.

- **Snack on healthy foods.** Snacking got a bad rap in the past by diet gurus who never found a snack they liked. In the past decade, that has changed; and the research shows that snacking between meals can actually be good for you, as long as you're smart about what you eat. The best snacks are high in energy like fruit, nuts, low-fat yogurt, and whole grain cereals.

- **Don't ignore minerals.** The only part of our diet that isn't created by a living organism is minerals, which we need even more than we do the vitamins that get much of the attention. Minerals are what make enzymes work, they help build cells, and they maintain and revitalize organ systems. Without good calcium levels, for example, our skeletal, nervous, and muscular systems don't function properly. Without iron, we can't make the hemoglobin that carries our oxygen, and we develop anemia. Magnesium is involved in nerve transmission and reactions that help us fight stress. Zinc is an important component of many enzymes that sustain life processes by speeding up chemical reactions. By consuming proper amounts of minerals, especially when stress robs you of those minerals, your body will repair and heal itself naturally.

• **Include foods that boost immunity.** Studies on populations throughout the world have shown that foods can heal, and diets that prevent disease are typically high in whole grains, fruits, and vegetables and low in meats and saturated fats. People with the lowest rates of cancer, heart disease, and other common illnesses load up on what I call the best healing foods: apples, beans, broccoli, cabbage, carrots, cauliflower, fish such as salmon and tuna, garlic, grapes, nuts such as almonds and walnuts, onions, peppers, spinach, oranges, and tomatoes.

• **Eat foods that decrease inflammation.** According to the latest research, inflammation is one of the leading causes of human disease. To reduce inflammation significantly, there are a number of tried and true diet strategies: reduce saturated and trans-fats, eat lots of green leafy vegetables, drink green tea, and consume omega-3 fatty acids every day. The best sources of omega-3 are those with high amounts of EPA and DHA like wild salmon, sardines, tuna, flaxseed, and walnuts. Another option is to take two to four grams of fish oil each day.

• **Give supplements a try.** Though the FDA and USDA have issued warnings on various toxic herbs and supplements, some others have been shown to be effective in boosting energy levels, increasing metabolism, strengthening immunity, and helping fight cancer and other diseases.

Supplement	Benefits and Potential Benefits
Apple Cider Vinegar	Helps regulate blood sugar, blood pressure, and cholesterol levels as well as eliminate toxins from the body. In order to get these benefits, the vinegar must be the raw, organic kind, not distilled and filtered. Make sure you take it with a full glass of water.
Astragalus	May boost immunity, improve kidney function, and stimulate red blood cell production.
Cayenne	Increases blood flow and therefore improves circulation and transport of oxygen to vital organs.
Cinnamon	Has been shown to lower blood pressure and blood sugar levels as well as LDL.
DHEA	May boost immunity, improves memory, elevates mood, relieves stress, and may protect against heart disease and atherosclerosis.
Fish Oil	The omega-3 in fish oil decreases inflammation, lowers cholesterol and triglycerides, and improves brain function. Make sure the label contains the amounts of EPA and DHA in the fish oil since these are the essential fatty acids that provide all the health benefits. Physicians for Optimal Heart and Brain Health recommend an EPA vs. DHA ratio of 2:1.
Flax Seed	Helps fight diabetes, reduces cholesterol, and decreases inflammation. Because it contains omega-3 fatty acids, it also helps fight heart disease.
Garlic	Improves cardiovascular health, lowers blood pressure, strengthens the immune system, and may have a powerful antioxidant effect, which protects against cancer.
Ginseng	Improves mental activity, combats fatigue, boosts energy levels, and strengthens the heart and nervous systems.
Green Tea	Has been shown to improve blood flow and lower cholesterol. A 2013 review of many studies found green tea helped prevent a range of heart-related issues, from high blood pressure to congestive heart failure. Green tea has also been shown to help block the formation of plaques that are linked to Alzheimer's disease.

Supplement	Benefits and Potential Benefits
Psyllium fiber	Lowers LDL, improves digestion, helps regulate blood pressure, and may reduce the risk of colon cancer.
Rhodiola	Can help improve mood, combat stress, and promote health neurotransmitter function.
Saw Palmetto	Reduces symptoms of enlarged prostate, strengthens the immune system, and helps relaxation by calming the nervous system.
Spirulina	Called nature's perfect food, spirulina is high in nutrients and antioxidants, and has been shown to cleanse the liver and eliminate toxins. It also helps reduce blood pressure and cholesterol and boosts the immune system.
Turmeric	The primary agent in turmeric, curcumin, has potent anti-inflammatory properties similar to many drugs and over-the-counter medications. It also has antioxidants that may help fight cancer and other diseases.

Rules for Buying Herbal Supplements

Consumers need to be aware that herbal supplements are not regulated; and though they are required to include an accurate label, they are not required to go through the FDA approval process. Therefore, some may be effective, but others may cause serious harm and sometimes death. Following these six guidelines before buying is always a wise thing to do.

- Ask yourself, "Does it sound too good to be true?" If the claims seem exaggerated or unrealistic, chances are they are. Learn to distinguish hype from evidence-based science, which involves a body of research, not a single study. Nonsensical lingo can sound convincing, so be skeptical about anecdotal information from slick salespeople who have no formal training in nutrition. Never buy a product just because it's touted as a miracle cure. Always question people about their training and knowledge in medicine or nutrition; and never assume that even if a product may not help, at least it can't hurt.

- Never assume that "natural" means healthy and safe. Consumers often think that the term natural assures wholesomeness, or that the product has milder effects, which makes it safer to use than a drug. The claim that something is natural can often be unsubstantiated. Herbs picked from a garden are natural, but they may interact with drugs or may be dangerous for people with certain medical conditions. What most consumers don't realize is that even groups that test herbal supplements, such as Good Housekeeping and NSF International, are not obligated to report products that don't meet their standards.

- Check for standardization. Since herbs are not regulated, they can vary in quality and content from one manufacturer to the next. The way an herb is grown, stored, prepared, and packaged will affect its potency and efficacy. Standardized herbs have been checked for uniformity, contaminants, and cleanliness. Never buy an herbal supplement that doesn't include a label with the active ingredient per given weight. And only buy "single herb" products that clearly indicate how much of the herb each dose contains. Avoid products that contain mixtures of herbs, since the proportion of each herb is generally unknown.

- Choose retailers and manufacturers wisely. Nothing on store shelves, especially health food stores, is created equally. While the FDA issues warnings about herbal supplements, it's up to consumers to educate themselves about the benefits and dangers of herbs. Therefore, it's especially important to choose retailers that are highly reputable and have the best-known brands. When browsing, read labels, look for standardization information, and make sure that the product you're buying has been scientifically tested. When buying from websites, be extra diligent about doing your homework.

- Use the proper herbal form. Everyone reacts to herbs differently, and much research has gone into determining the formulations herbs need to be in for maximum effectiveness. Some herbs are best absorbed if they're in liquid or gel form, others are fat-soluble and most effective as tablets. Herbs are also metabolized differently in children and adults, so a safe dose for an adult may not be for children who are under eighteen. Reputable stores have a knowledgeable sales staff and the experience to know which herbal supplements should be taken by whom and in which forms.

- Be aware of interactions. Like foods, herbs can interact with prescription drugs, as well as with other herbal supplements. Always consult your doctor before taking any herbal product; and when asked if you're taking anything, always tell your doctor exactly which herbs you're using. According to the Mayo Clinic, the medications that interact with herbs most are: blood pressure medicines, blood thinners, diabetes medications, drugs that affect the liver, heart medications, and monoamine oxidase inhibitors. Stop taking an herb immediately if you notice any adverse side effect at all.

Food and Stress

What we eat has a direct effect on how we feel, how we cope with stressful life events, and how well we maintain our immune systems. Foods high in saturated fats, like red meats, and refined sugar, like white bread, cause us to produce more insulin. More insulin means less fat breakdown, as well as a bigger appetite, which leads to overeating. Some foods, called "high stress foods," can make stress worse; others can actually help us combat stress and keep us healthy during those times when we need it most.

- **Foods That May Increase Stress Effects**
  Cake, candy, cold cuts (except for low-fat meats such as turkey and chicken breast), doughnuts, fried foods, meats high in saturated fat, sweet rolls, white pasta, white rice, whole milk, white bread

- **Foods That May Reduce Stress Effects**
  Beans, brown rice, chicken breast (not fried), cottage cheese, fat-free or low-fat milk, fish, fruit (especially apples, bananas, cantaloupe, oranges, and pineapple), legumes, nuts, oatmeal, soybeans, sunflower seeds, turkey breast, vegetables (especially dark green and those with beta-carotene), wheat germ, whole grain cereal, whole wheat bread.

Carbohydrate Cycling

The more body fat you store, especially around the midsection, the more your hormone levels will be affected and the greater your risk becomes of developing disease. Since the brain is linked to virtually every bodily function, and hormones play a key role in both mental and physical health, losing those extra pounds around the middle will certainly keep the mind-body connection healthy as well.

Carbohydrate cycling has been used by bodybuilders for decades as a way to burn fat quickly and to show off their muscles. It has always been a kind of secret weapon during competition season when they needed to get their total body fat as low as possible. After all, you can have all the muscle in the world, but if there's a layer of body fat covering it, what good does it do? But, carb cycling isn't just for bodybuilders; it's for people who want to reduce their carbohydrate input and maintain a healthy weight.

To cycle, all you need to do is alternate high-carb days that boost metabolism with low-carb days that break down fat and build muscle. On high-carb days, eat plenty of fruits, vegetables, whole wheat breads, pasta, and whole grains, in addition to protein at every meal. Minimize fats on these days. On low-carb days, consume protein and good fats but very few carbs, except for breakfast. Regardless of which day you're on, always eat three meals and two healthy snacks per day every three hours to maintain metabolism and keep from getting hungry. And remember to eat protein at every meal. On the seventh day, reward yourself by eating anything you want before starting the cycle again.

The Curative Properties of Water

Two-thirds of the human body is made up of water. When your body loses 2 percent of its total fluid, you begin to experience the symptoms of dehydration. Even a slight loss of body fluids affects the brain; and we know the extent to which the brain controls the rest of the body. Some of the more common effects are thirst, loss of appetite, dry skin, dark urine, dry mouth, and fatigue. Fluid loss of 5 percent leads to increased heart rate and respiration, decreased perspiration and higher body temperature, extreme fatigue, and muscle cramps. A loss of 10 percent is so severe that dehydration becomes an emergency that must be treated immediately.

Each of us reacts differently to dehydration because we're all unique. Age, size, and health all play a role in how we react physically, but not drinking enough water can lead to some common disorders we normally don't think of as being caused by dehydration. For example:

- **High blood pressure:** Blood loses gases as water leaves the circulatory system and, therefore, blood vessels constrict in order to prevent further loss.

- **High cholesterol:** One of the main components of cell membranes is cholesterol. As a defense mechanism, the body increases the production of cholesterol in order to keep cells from dehydrating.

- **High blood sugar:** When blood volume decreases as a result of dehydration, circulation through the capillaries decreases and the concentration of blood sugar rises in relation to other blood chemicals.

- **Decreased muscle building:** Muscles need water for protein synthesis. When there's not enough water, muscle fibers begin to break down and strength levels decline.

- **Increased joint pain:** Water is a major component of cartilage in the body, which includes joints. It also carries the nutrients that help build cartilage and prevent inflammation, abrasion and wear and tear. Furthermore, because water is stored in the vertebrae, it acts to support the weight of the upper body and prevent back pain.

- **Increased buildup of toxins:** The kidney is the body's natural dialysis system, filtering the entire blood supply and removing toxins from the body. A good fluid level will keep the kidneys functioning properly and help the body rid itself of toxic substances.

You can see how drinking adequate amounts of water can prevent the onset of many disorders and keep your mind and body in a state of balance. But unless you're exercising vigorously or working out in the sun, you don't need to drink eight glasses of water a day as some health gurus claim. Many of the foods and liquids we drink have enough water to keep us hydrated. A good way to gauge how dehydrated you are is to look at the color of your urine. If it's clear or a very pale yellow, it's a good sign that you're hydrated. If it begins to turn dark, you need to drink more. That's all there is to it.

Is Sugar Toxic?

Recent evidence about sugar and how much of it we consume is painting a sobering picture of how sugar is linked to a number of diseases such as diabetes, heart disease, hypertension, and cancer. Until a few years ago, the main dietary culprit was fat. But to the surprise of researchers, as fat was replaced with sugar in many products, the incidence of heart disease went up, not down. The average weight of the population also went up. We now know that the simple sugars found in soda and other sugary drinks, cookies, and candies are also found in foods we might not even realize contain sugars, and are the main cause of the skyrocketing obesity and Type II diabetes epidemics.

According to Dr. Robert Lustig, a pediatric endocrinologist at the University of California, the amount of sugar and high fructose corn syrup in processed foods is creating an entire generation of obese and sick children. One of the main ways it's doing this is by increasing small dense LDL, the type of LDL cholesterol that clogs the arteries and leads to heart disease. And with the average person consuming nearly 130 pounds of sugar per year, the rates of disease will continue to increase.

One recent study, by Kimber Stanhope, PhD at the University of California–Davis, found that calories from sugar are different than calories from other foods. When subjects were given sweetened drinks as part of a controlled diet, their LDL cholesterol went up after just two weeks because the liver begins to convert the fructose into fat, which then gets into the bloodstream to create the small dense LDL molecules.[12]

Another study found that sugar actually helps certain types of cancer tumors grow.[13] Breast cancers and colon cancer, for example, contain insulin receptors, which allow the tumor to absorb sugar in the presence of insulin. When an individual with a tumor consumes too much sugar, the flood of insulin binds to the receptors on the cancer cell membrane and helps the tumor consume sugar. The result: the cancer feeds on the sugar and grows more rapidly. Nearly a third of all cancers contain these insulin receptors; so if an individual has a weakened immune system and develops a tumor, sugar may be the last thing he or she wants to consume.

Keeping the mind-body connection healthy means eating the right foods, taking the proper kinds and amounts of vitamins and minerals, avoiding certain supplements that can do more harm than good, living a wholesome lifestyle, and knowing how to read nutrition labels. Since proper nutrition boosts immunity and helps prevent illness and disease, the saying "we are what we eat" is truer than we may think. By avoiding unhealthy behaviors, being a responsible and knowledgeable consumer, and taking a proactive approach to our health, we'll maximize the potential for a healthy immune system well into old age.

CHAPTER FOUR

Conditioning the Brain to Prevent Illness

There's not a disease or illness in the world that is not, in one way or another, affected, intensified, or triggered by stress. From the common cold to cancer, every disease begins with a breakdown in immunity and homeostasis, which then triggers even further attacks on the immune system. The disease progresses until it's either eliminated by natural defenses or medication(s), or thrives and overwhelms the body's organ systems. One of the most significant contributing factors in the latter process is physical or emotional stress.

Long before humans ever thought about stress, our early ancestors depended on the stress response for their survival. Fleeing predators, fighting enemies, and surviving a hostile world didn't leave much room for the weak and helpless. Those able to respond to life-threatening events survived and passed their genes on to their offspring. Those who could not eventually died off.

With each generation, the ability to respond to stress increased and evolved to what it is today: an amazingly efficient and complex set of reactions that protect us during times of emergency, but when left unchecked can make us sick and trigger a variety of illnesses. The origin of modern stress, then, has its roots in our primitive past. What began as a vital defense mechanism has morphed into the leading cause of disease and illness in the modern world. And as society becomes ever more complex, and every succeeding generation is forced to cope with new kinds of stressors, we're finding that more and more people are falling victim to stress-related health disorders.

Stress Begins in the Brain

Stress is categorized as acute or chronic, physical or emotional. Anyone who's ever experienced intense physical trauma knows exactly what physical stress can do to health and well-being. Interestingly, studies have found that, in terms of overall effect on the body, emotional or psychological stress can be even more damaging than physical stress. But regardless of the type of stress the human body encounters, especially if it's long-term or chronic, the impact on organ systems is profound. During stress, powerful signals from the brain and the nervous system either stimulate or inhibit various physiological functions. And by interfering with important chemical pathways, stress blocks the body's production of white blood cells, which then inhibits immunity.

One of the main reasons stress affects us so much is that virtually every organ system in our body reacts in a collective effort to protect us from whatever triggered stress in the first place. It's the classic "fight or flight" response that served our ancestors so well in the past and today continues to help us in emergency situations. But the body doesn't recognize nuances or variations of stress; it simply interprets the brain's message that we have encountered some sort of "threat" and must mobilize to deal with it.

Everyone differs in what they view as stressful or potentially stressful. But the main causes of stress are the same: fear, both physical and psychological; uncertainty about life events, resources, finances, and situations; negative perceptions and attitudes regarding work, home-life, society, etc.; and change, whether it's positive or negative.

The brain and the immune system are in constant communication, in a delicate balance that can be thrown off by chronic stress. The hypothalamus plays a key role in the stress response, releasing corticotropin-releasing hormone (CRH), which stimulates the pituitary gland to release another hormone, adrenocorticotropic hormone (ACTH), into the bloodstream. ACTH then causes the adrenal glands to release cortisol. In addition to alerting the body to meet stressful situations, cortisol helps regulate the immune system. The hypothalamus uses both cortisol and special molecules from the immune system called cytokines to monitor the body and ensure that there isn't an immune system overreaction that harms healthy cells and tissues. Problems anywhere along the system can lead to disease.

Basically, two things happen during the classic stress response: (1) the brain's hypothalamus sends nerve impulses to the pituitary and the adrenal glands, and (2) the rest of the nervous system is stimulated to either trigger or inhibit responses from the rest of the body's organs, tissues, and glands. In concert, this cascade of events is what we feel whenever we're stressed.

Though the stress response is a series of biochemical and physiological events that provide our body with the biological ammunition needed to maintain homeostatic mechanisms, three overriding reactions occur: (1) a massive surge of adrenaline, (2) a sudden discharge of cortisol, and (3) a release of endorphin. Let's look at each of these molecules to see exactly why it is that we feel and act the way we do during stress.

Adrenaline: Adrenaline, or epinephrine, stimulates the autonomic nervous system. A surge of adrenaline causes heart rate, blood pressure, breathing rate, and metabolism to increase. These events bring needed oxygen and nutrients to the tissues and brain. Oxygen is nature's purest fuel, driving our biochemical reactions, regulating blood gases such as carbon dioxide, and pumping extra energy into our system. Adrenaline also causes the blood vessels within the skeletal muscles to dilate and carry additional materials to certain parts of the body while causing other blood vessels within the digestive system to constrict in order for more blood to be shunted to muscle.

To boost energy levels during stress, adrenaline causes an increase in glucose by breaking down glycogen in the liver and an increase in free fatty acids by breaking down lipids in adipose tissue. Glycogen, the stored form of sugar in humans, is converted to glucose by a remarkable set of reactions that produce billions of glucose molecules within seconds of a stress reaction, thus providing us with an instant source of vital energy. Adrenalin also triggers bronchodilation for enhanced breathing capacity to deliver extra oxygen (asthma sufferers, for example, inhale epinephrine drugs to open air passages in the lungs).

Cortisol: Produced by the cortex or outer layer of the adrenal gland, cortisol has widespread effects on the body in terms of metabolism and immunity. The first thing our body does when it encounters stress is to make sure that any damage done to cells and tissues is repaired. Cortisol, therefore, breaks down proteins and ensures that we have enough circulating amino acids to make new protein and repair injured tissue. Other physiologic effects of cortisol are to break down lipids into fatty acids and glycogen into glucose for increased energy and to decrease inflammation and allergic reactions by preventing the release of histamines.

While cortisol is essential for life, over-secretion will ultimately lead to illness and disease. As we saw earlier, stress-induced cortisol release leads to decreased production of white blood cells, natural killer (NK) cells, and antibodies. Chronic stress, therefore, possesses one of the greatest risks for increasing vulnerability to contracting a host of illnesses and diseases.

Endorphin: We're all familiar with the term "runner's high," a condition in which an athlete becomes almost euphoric after thirty minutes of beginning his or her run. Known as the body's natural tranquilizer, endorphin or "endogenous morphine" is an opioid (exhibits opiate-like qualities) produced by the brain and the pituitary gland. Stress or intense physical activity triggers release of endorphin with subsequent analgesia or blockage of pain.

Drugs such as opioid pain medications, along with heroin, opium, and morphine, bind to the same opioid receptors as endorphin does because they all have similar molecular structures. They block pain by attaching to receptors in an area of the brain that processes pain perception. Because of this, individuals are effectively able to block pain by triggering release of beta-endorphin through such activities as electric stimulation, acupuncture, and exercise.

But, just as adrenaline and cortisol produce negative effects in their effort to combat stress, endorphin has its dark side as well. Too much endorphin depresses immune function and NK activity and decreases testosterone and estrogen levels. In the short term, it serves us well as an analgesic; but in the end, continued release of endorphins makes us more susceptible to illness and disease and significantly interferes with sexual function and reproduction.

Any effective stress management strategy has as its basic foundation the principle that in order to eliminate negative stress reactions and relieve stress, one must first condition the brain. Stress reactions, in many cases triggered as a result of conditioning and negative habit formation, can be eliminated by using the power of the brain to break those habits.

Test Your Coping Skills

How well do you think you cope with stress? The following stress scale was developed by the Public Health Service of the US Department of Health and Human Services, largely on the basis of results compiled by clinicians and researchers who tried to identify how people effectively cope with stress. It's an educational tool, designed to help inform you of the most effective and healthy ways to cope.

_____ Give yourself 10 points if you feel you have supportive family around you.

_____ Give yourself 10 points if you actively pursue a hobby.

_____ Give yourself 10 points if you belong to a social or activity group in which you participate more than once a month.

_____ Give yourself 15 points if you are within 10 pounds of your "ideal" body weight, considering your height and bone structure.

_____ Give yourself 15 points if you practice some form of "deep relaxation" at least five times a week. Deep relaxation includes meditation, progressive muscle relaxation, imagery, and yoga.

_____ Give yourself 5 points for each time you exercise for thirty minutes or longer during an average week.

_____ Give yourself 5 points for each nutritionally balanced and wholesome meal you eat during an average day. A nutritionally balanced meal is low in fat and high in vegetables, fruits, and whole-grain products.

_____ Give yourself 5 points if you do something you really enjoy and that is "just for you" during an average week.

_____ Give yourself 10 points if you have a place in your home to which you can go to relax or be by yourself.

_____ Give yourself 10 points if you practice time management techniques daily.

_____ Subtract 10 points for each pack of cigarettes you smoke during an average day.

_____ Subtract 5 points for each evening during an average week that you use any form of medication or chemical substance, including alcohol, to help you sleep.

_____ Subtract 10 points for each day during an average week that you consume any form of medication or chemical substance, including alcohol, to reduce anxiety or just to calm down.

_____ Subtract 5 points for each evening during an average week that you bring work home—work meant to be done at your place of employment.

_____ **Total**

A perfect score is 115. If you scored 50–60, you have adequate coping skills for most common stress. The higher your score, the greater your ability to cope with stress in a healthy manner.

Stress Response as a Conditioned Habit

A habit is defined as a behavior pattern that becomes regular or spontaneous as a result of repetition. It becomes stronger and easier to trigger over time because it gets ingrained in our subconscious and is released as a conditioned response whenever we're exposed to a specific mental or environmental cue. This conditioning process is influenced by what we learn, how we act, and how often we do the things we do whenever we encounter events that trigger the response. The longer the conditioning occurs and the stronger the habit becomes, the more difficult it is to reverse the trend.

From the moment we're born, we become creatures of habit. For the most part, that's a good thing. Habits free our minds of routine tasks and simplify our day-to-day existence. We rely on them to accomplish what would otherwise require thought and preparation. As children, writing, tying shoelaces, and even eating with utensils are the direct results of habit formation. Later in life, more complex tasks are greatly simplified because we do them without thinking. Habits, therefore, are an important part of life in that they allow us to function more efficiently.

The problem occurs when we begin to acquire habits regardless of whether they're good or bad, positively or negatively reinforced. Our body doesn't make the distinction. It simply becomes conditioned through a subconscious mechanism that's reinforced through repetition. Stress is no different. And just like any habit that becomes ingrained until it is part and parcel of our everyday life, the stress habit becomes a conditioned response that needs to be broken before it gets out of hand and causes illness. Here's a classic example I always use:

John gets a new job and soon becomes irritated at the way his boss is treating him. Since he needs the job, he can't do anything about it for fear of getting fired. Every time he has a confrontation with his boss, John has a stress response. His heart rate and blood pressure go up, he feels himself becoming tense, and his stomach is tied up in knots. The reactions begin to come more easily, more quickly, and are of longer duration with each encounter. Eventually, the mere thought of a confrontation triggers stress reactions. He soon experiences these negative reactions at home and on weekends by just thinking about his boss. In the end, John's stress response becomes a major habit that gets progressively worse and harder to break.

Like John, if we don't do anything about our situation, if we allow ourselves to become conditioned to the point that we respond merely at the thought of being stressed out, we'll plunge into a vicious cycle that's typical of job stress and burnout. The more we encounter stress, the more we begin to think about it, even when we're not stressed. And the more we think about it, the more intensely we respond to it and the more easily we condition ourselves to respond to it the next time. One of the best ways to reverse this pattern is through behavior modification techniques that transform negative thoughts into positive and constructive attitudes. I'll give examples later in the chapter.

Chronic stress response, whether it occurs as a result of our job or anything else, is the end product of a runaway conditioning process. And like any other bad habit, it too needs to be controlled through changes in behavior, attitude, and lifestyle. By conditioning ourselves to spontaneously relax, to relieve tension, to cope with conflict, and to eliminate anxiety, we'll gain freedom from stress and improve the quality of our lives.

Stress Rating Scale[14]

In terms of body chemistry, we all respond to stressful events in the same way. But the degree of our physiological responses and the extent to which we're affected are different across individuals. That's because each of us perceives things in a different way. What's stressful for you may not be for someone else. According to Drs. Thomas Holmes and Richard Rahe, there are certain life events that are universally stressful for people regardless of whether those events are perceived as positive or negative. A vacation, for instance, may be a wonderful way to relax and get away from it all, but for some it may be dreadful in that it involves planning, organization, and preparation. So, even pleasant changes and experiences can create stress, trigger stress reactions, and depress immunity.

Together, Drs. Holmes and Rahe developed a scale that ranks various stressors according to their intensity and severity. Their research has shown that experiencing stress events adding up to more than 300 points during any one year can lead to stress-related illness and disease. Some of the events may be perceived as more or as less severe than others by different individuals, but on average they're fairly consistent. The following is adapted from their research:

Event	Scale of Impact
Death of spouse	100
Divorce	73
Marital separation	65
Jail term	63
Death of family member	63
Personal injury or illness	53
Marriage	50
Fired from your job	47
Retirement	45
Change in the health of family member	44
Pregnancy	40
Sexual dysfunction	39
Adding a new family member	39
Change in financial state	38
Death of a close friend	37
Change in careers	36
Foreclosure of mortgage or loan	30
Change in work responsibilities	29
Son or daughter leaving home	29
Trouble with in-laws	29
Outstanding personal achievement	28
Spouse begins or stops work	26
Begin or end school	26
Change in living conditions	25
Change in personal habits	24
Conflicts with boss	23
Change in work hours or conditions	20
Change in residence	20

Change in schools	20
Change in recreational activities	19
Change in church activities	19
Change in social activities	18
Change in sleeping habits	16
Change in number of family gatherings	15
Change in eating habits	15
Vacation	13
Christmas	12
Minor violations of the law	11

There's no easy way to predict how much stress is too much because stressors often work together to magnify our response and increase its intensity. The stress response, then, is really a group of physiological reactions set off during any kind of stress event. Factors such as diet, genes, and lifestyle just multiply stress effects and complicate the picture even more.

The mind essentially perceives every event we encounter, processes it, and causes us to respond, in some cases in a way that increases the likelihood of disease. As a short-term defense mechanism, the stress response is a critical part of life. Our goal, however, should be to condition our brain so that (a) we don't over-respond and cause chronic health problems, and (b) that we maintain our immune system in order to help us fight off illness and disease whenever we need to.

How Stress Affects Weight

Gaining weight has a lot to do with genetics, eating foods high in fat and simple sugars, inactivity, and a sedentary lifestyle. Often overlooked in weight gain, however, is the effect that stress hormones have on appetite and on how fat is deposited in our body. Cortisol, the main stress hormone, triggers weight gain due to its effect on insulin, carbohydrate metabolism, satiety, and fat cells. Here is the series of events related to weight that occur whenever we encounter stress:

- The brain's pituitary gland releases ACTH, which stimulates the adrenal glands to produce the stress hormone cortisol.

- Cortisol breaks down glycogen, the body's stored form of carbohydrate, into simple sugar molecules needed for energy. It also stimulates the release of excess insulin, which adds to the problem by causing the body to store even more fat and inhibiting the breakdown of fat for energy.

- Both cortisol and insulin stimulate the brain's appetite center, so we keep eating. And since the main function of insulin is to allow cells to absorb sugar, the more sugar they absorb the less fat the body thinks it needs to break down.

- Stress inhibits the hormone leptin, which is normally secreted by fat cells to suppress appetite and increase metabolism. Without leptin, we continue eating but are not burning off the extra calories.

- The combination of ACTH, cortisol, insulin, and decreased leptin can make us fat quickly.

Unfortunately, the stressful life events that are responsible for so many health problems are also a factor in weight gain. The bright side is that controlling stress will also help us fight the battle of the bulge—another good reason to use stress management techniques.

Developing Stress Tolerance

Can stress actually energize us? Can it help us work better, or keep us healthier? Is there such a thing as good stress? And if so, is it possible to transform bad stress into good stress? The answer to all these questions is a resounding yes!

How we handle stress is determined by age, intelligence, education, income, religion, previous experiences, and personality type. As important as these factors are, conditioning, attitude, behavior, and habit formation have an equally profound effect on how the mind perceives and the body responds. Thus, experiences and life events can be either good or bad depending on how well we become "stress-tolerant," i.e., how well we can alter our attitudes and behaviors in order to condition our brain to look at stress in a new and different way. Figure 4.1 illustrates how perceptions affect immunity.

Figure 4.1: Effects of Perceptions on Conditioned Immune Responses

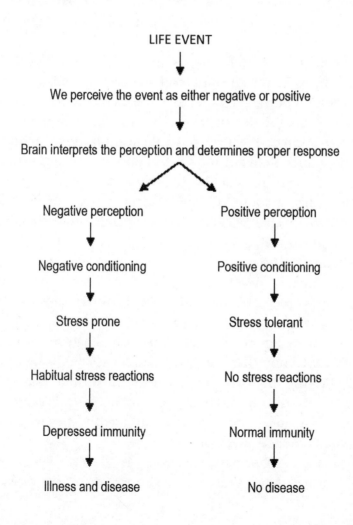

The same conditioning process used in triggering stress reactions can be used to change our response to stress from one that's negative and harmful to one that's actually positive and beneficial. By using certain mental images, exercises, and self-instructions, we can recondition ourselves to view stress as constructive rather than destructive. Stress-tolerant individuals, rather than trying to avoid stress, use it to overcome obstacles, meet challenges head on, and enhance the quality of their lives by responding to stress as a positive force that energizes and makes them more productive. Those who've succeeded in becoming stress-tolerant have done so by conditioning themselves to take negative situations and turn them into positive events.

Becoming stress-tolerant is basically conditioned or learned. In order to transform bad stress into good, we must first condition ourselves to perceive things differently than we have in the past. Since the mind controls the body, how we think has a direct effect on physiological reactions. Without exception, stress-tolerant individuals possess certain attitudes toward life that include having control over events and situations, being committed and having a sense of purpose, being open to change, and viewing change as a challenge rather than a threat.

To illustrate how the same stress is perceived differently, causing different reactions, studies were done on three groups of people. One study done with nurses showed that non-intensive care nurses experienced much higher levels of anxiety, reported more physical ailments, and had greater work load dissatisfaction than intensive care nurses did. It was later found that the intensive care nurses wanted more challenge and felt more adventurous than their counterparts. Because the intensive care nurses perceived stress differently, they were able to minimize anxiety and distress.

In a study of business executives, it was discovered that the executives who remained healthiest and most disease-free during their careers were the ones who had a sense of commitment, felt in control of their lives, and sought novelty and change rather than familiarity. They viewed change as an opportunity and a challenge; and when stress occurred, they became enthusiastic and energized instead of worried and depressed.

Finally, when a group of lawyers was studied, it was found that those who were seen as least stressed were often the ones who became physically sick the most often—exactly the opposite of what was expected. After looking more closely at how these lawyers were trained during law school, it became clear why this happened. Lawyers are conditioned to believe that they perform best under pressure. This perception of stress as a performance-enhancer allows them to deal with it as a non-threatening and even beneficial phenomenon. In this case, their conditioning made them believe that stress brought out the best in them and, therefore, they responded differently than most of us would.

Mind-Body Suggestions for Stress Tolerance

In the previous chapter, I described some practical ways to alter behavior in order to condition the brain to become less susceptible to stress-related illness. But to become more stress-tolerant, we need to develop a new mindset. A good way to do that is to use mental suggestions and the power of the mind to instill in ourselves a more stress-tolerant attitude. After all, stress tolerance begins in the brain at the very moment we pick up a stress signal and respond to it in a specific way.

Using mind-body suggestions as a normal daily routine accomplishes an important goal: it conditions our brain to think differently about stress. Once we change our negative mindset and perceive stress as a challenge, we begin to take charge of situations rather than allowing them to take charge of us. This is the basic principle behind stress tolerance. Learning to eliminate negative thoughts will subconsciously turn bad stress into the catalyst that enables us to become more positive and constructive in the way we approach whatever we do.

The mind-body suggestions I teach in my seminars should be used in the same way you would use the technique of autohypnosis. By reading or saying them out loud each day for a few weeks, the conditioning process becomes more powerful. Before you know it, these suggestions will automatically be ingrained as part of your day-to-day subconscious and become incorporated into normal thought processes. Once they're wired into your brain, they'll become a spontaneous and natural response to any kind of stress event. Here are my favorites:

When I commit to something and get involved, I have a feeling of accomplishment and strength.

By committing to something, whatever it is, we feel a sense of worth and purpose. Most of us tend to be passive rather than active by nature. Being actively involved and committed gives direction and meaning to our lives, and we begin to lose our negative attitudes. By telling ourselves that our activity and involvement is a positive experience, we'll have a better outlook on life, feel better about ourselves in general, and begin to experience fewer negative stress reactions.

Change is exciting and rewarding.

Most of us view change in our lives as something negative. More often than not, we allow change to occur without making an effort to transform it into a positive experience. Sometimes we just get complacent about change, and that only causes us to have little if any feeling of excitement. To counter this, get into the habit of viewing any kind of change as positive, challenging, exciting, and rewarding.

Whenever I take charge, I get a feeling of power that energizes me.

Having a sense of control is one of the key factors in our ability to transform negative stress into a positive situation. Negative stress isn't caused by job pressures and negative events but rather by the feelings we have that what we do is not worthwhile and that most things are beyond our control. The result is often burnout, which then leads to illness and disease. Having a sense of control over a situation energizes us and helps channel that energy into constructive activities. By involving ourselves and being committed to what we're doing, we automatically develop a sense of control that conditions the brain to think in a new way. In turn, this causes us to behave differently and to change our attitudes and perceptions. In no time at all, we realize that we'd rather control than be controlled.

Stress makes me productive and worthwhile.
Rather than allowing stress to beat you, visualize it energizing you instead. Stress can actually boost your performance and make you reach your full potential. Just as champion athletes perform best when they're under pressure, and world records are typically broken when the best athletes are competing against each other, most people rise to a higher level when they're challenged. Your body will respond to what your brain is conditioned to perceive; so if you get into the habit of thinking like an athlete, rather than causing grief and fatigue, stress will bring out the best in us.

Type A vs. Type B Personality

Attitude is the mental processes used to respond to stimuli. Personality is the sum total of habitual physical and mental activities, attitudes, interests, and behaviors. It's who we are and what makes us different from anyone else. According to psychologists, each of us is molded into a unique individual during childhood and characterized by one of sixteen different personality types. Based on recent studies, having a certain personality type could make us more prone to illness and disease.

When heart disease became one of the world's leading killers, it was assumed that anyone leading a stressful lifestyle or having certain behavioral traits was at risk. Certain individuals were seen as more susceptible to coronary heart disease, cancer, and other stress-related illnesses. Individuals having this behavior pattern, or Type A personality, were shown to have at least some of the following general characteristics:

- Increased muscle gestures, such as grimaces, teeth grinding, and jaw clenching
- Time urgency and impatience; frustration if things are not done quickly
- More intense response to stress; increased heart rate and blood pressure
- Worried about finishing tasks and accomplishing goals
- Competitive and highly achievement-oriented
- Ambitious and driven to succeed at all costs
- Need to be productive; feel guilty when not
- Strong need to be in charge or in control
- Preoccupied with what to do "next"
- Need to be recognized
- Always seem rushed

Many people ask, "Is there such a thing as a healthy Type A?" The answer depends on the extent and intensity of the behavior. If your behavior is so competitive and aggressive that it leads to anger and hostility, it's considered the "toxic" factor in Type A personality, and then the answer is no. Sometimes an individual who is mildly Type A begins to exhibit more and more of the toxic traits and becomes a full-fledged Type A individual who is then at greater risk of disease. So it's difficult to be a healthy Type A unless you adopt some Type B personality traits.

Some years ago, a group of cardiologists observed certain behaviors in their (predominantly) male coronary patients. Surprisingly, diet and cholesterol were not as high on their list as sociocultural influences and job stress. When their wives and coworkers were interviewed, the answers about the patients' behavior were the same, and they included many of the characteristics listed on page 86. It was the doctors' conclusion that risk factors like diet alone were often not enough to trigger heart disease. Type As, in their opinion, were heart patients because they exhibited classic Type A personality traits.

In contrast, Type B individuals are much more relaxed, less worried about time, less affected by stress, not as competitive or ambitious, and are not as driven or highly achievement-oriented. They view situations in a less intense manner, are better able to put things into perspective, and think through how they're going to deal with situations rather than reacting or flying off the handle. Consequently they tend to be less stress-prone and have a lower cardiovascular response to stress.

Type A Personality Quiz

The following is a Type A personality quiz I have been giving for years that should help assess your personality traits and behavioral type. Read each statement and then check the number corresponding to the category of behavior that best fits you (1 = never; 2 = seldom; 3 = sometimes; 4 = usually; 5 = always). After you finish, tally your score and compare it to the key at the end of the quiz.

	1	2	3	4	5
I become annoyed if I have to stand in line for more than fifteen minutes.	☐	☐	☐	☐	☐
I am a naturally competitive individual.	☐	☐	☐	☐	☐
I'm always looking for the next promotion or achievement.	☐	☐	☐	☐	☐
I can't seem to relax and take it easy.	☐	☐	☐	☐	☐
I find myself constantly networking with new people.	☐	☐	☐	☐	☐
I grow impatient when someone's talking too slowly.	☐	☐	☐	☐	☐

	1	2	3	4	5
I consider myself a perfectionist.	☐	☐	☐	☐	☐
I bring my laptop with me on vacation.	☐	☐	☐	☐	☐
I work best under pressure and deadlines.	☐	☐	☐	☐	☐
I bring work home with me on most work days.	☐	☐	☐	☐	☐
I'm a take charge person who likes to be in control.	☐	☐	☐	☐	☐
I find multitasking to be the best way to get things done.	☐	☐	☐	☐	☐
I'm usually at the center of a conversation.	☐	☐	☐	☐	☐
I don't usually take the time to do things for myself.	☐	☐	☐	☐	☐
I get angry when I lose at sports or other competitions.	☐	☐	☐	☐	☐
I'm constantly looking at my watch.	☐	☐	☐	☐	☐
I eat rapidly in order to get back to work.	☐	☐	☐	☐	☐
I feel rushed, even when I have plenty of time to get things done.	☐	☐	☐	☐	☐
I get bored easily.	☐	☐	☐	☐	☐
I never seem to have time for a vacation.	☐	☐	☐	☐	☐
I micromanage at work and at home.	☐	☐	☐	☐	☐
I prefer when things are done quickly.	☐	☐	☐	☐	☐
I think about work, even when I'm trying to relax.	☐	☐	☐	☐	☐
I'm not very flexible when it comes to change.	☐	☐	☐	☐	☐
I find that stress energizes me.	☐	☐	☐	☐	☐
I grow impatient when things are not done the way I think they should be.	☐	☐	☐	☐	☐
I'm usually the first one to finish dinner at a restaurant.	☐	☐	☐	☐	☐
I find myself arguing with people who don't work as hard as I do.	☐	☐	☐	☐	☐

	1 2 3 4 5
I spend part of my weekends finishing up work projects.	☐ ☐ ☐ ☐ ☐
I consider myself more serious than most people.	☐ ☐ ☐ ☐ ☐

The minimum score is 30, the maximum 150. The breakdown by personality type is as follows:

SCORE	PERSONALITY TYPE
100–150	Type A
76–99	Type AB (Average)
30–75	Type B

Since each of us is unique, and we react to life events in different ways—there *are* no correct or incorrect answers. Spending the weekend working on a project or getting ready for next week's meeting may be stressful for you, but someone else may find it exciting and exhilarating. And Type Bs can be just as productive and equally as efficient as Type As. There comes a point, however, when too many of those Type A behavior patterns begin to take their toll and lead to health problems. And that's when adopting some Type B traits can be a good thing.

Every Type A has some Type B personality traits and vice versa. However, Type B or Type AB behavior is beneficial to your health because it allows you to function productively and achieve your goals without resorting to the negative Type A behaviors like competitiveness, impatience, and aggression. By conditioning yourself to think and act more like a Type B individual, you'll make your life easier, more enjoyable, and stress-free. In the process, you'll find that you feel better and get sick less often.

Behavior Modification for Type A

Because emotional factors often associated with Type A personality can have a powerful effect on the heart and other organs, it's easy to see why, as early as the nineteenth century, the German physician von Dusch first noted that excessive work was a hallmark of people who died from heart attacks. Later, in the twentieth century, several studies linked coronary patients with aggressive behavior, ambition, competitiveness, intense drive, and unrealistic goals. Today, psychologists use questionnaires like the Jenkins Activity Survey to help people detect Type A behavior because many individuals are either unaware of their Type A tendencies or deny them.

We become Type A or Type B because of genetics and environment. And since it's part and parcel of our genes and our personality, we can't just decide that we're going to become one or the other; all we can do is modify our existing behavior patterns so that we're more comfortable in a different skin so to speak. The more we practice Type B behaviors, the easier they become and the more our brain is conditioned to accept them.

So the key to Type A behavior modification is using the mind-body connection and brain conditioning to break habits formed over a lifetime. We essentially form new habits that replace the old, unhealthy ones. Some of us may not even be Type A to begin with, but because of jobs, life situations, and upbringing, we've taken on Type A traits and simply assume we're Type A when we really aren't.

The following behavior modification exercises are a great way to start breaking Type A habits. The more you practice them, the more ingrained they'll become and the more natural they'll feel. It's important to do these and not just think about them because physically doing something is a more powerful brain conditioner than mentally visualizing doing something. In just a few weeks, you'll be well on your way to modifying the habits that are putting you at risk.

- **Try acting in the opposite way.** Deliberately change your normal behavior pattern. If you talk more than you listen, force yourself to pay attention to what people are saying and just listen more. If you find yourself irritated and impatient while waiting in line, for example, make a conscientious effort to think about something else, smile, or start a conversation with the person in line with you.

- **Force yourself to slow down.** For the next few weeks, do everything as if you were in lower gear. Eat slower, chew slower, walk a little slower to your car or office, listen quietly to the conversations of other people without interrupting, and stop on occasion to "smell the flowers."

- **Plan relaxing activities.** Make a list of activities to do that are not work-related or too over-stimulating. Learn the meditation and relaxation techniques in this book and then practice them daily, even if it's for ten minutes.

- **Do more fun things.** Make an effort to read more novels, see more fun movies, take walks, eat out, go on vacation, and do the things you enjoy doing but never seem to fit into your schedule. Sometimes it's a matter of prioritizing; sometimes it is as simple as just doing it.

- **Leave your watch at home.** Time urgency is not an exclusively Type A personality trait. Even Type B gets in the habit of constantly being concerned about time. By spending an entire day without your watch, you'll free yourself from one of the worst Type A behaviors and realize how nice it is not to be a clock watcher.

- **Talk to yourself in a positive way.** Remind yourself every day that life is good and that you're luckier than most. When things seem to be going wrong, stop, take a few breaths, and just say, "Relax, take it easy, it's going to be okay." Hearing yourself say positive expressions will condition the brain to think that way. Before long it becomes automatic.

- **Reward yourself for achieving Type B goals.** Write down specific Type B goals, and then reward yourself for achieving them. It could be something as simple as treating yourself to a nice dinner out. The brain subconsciously links the reward with the modified behavior and strengthens the conditioning process.

By practicing Type B personality traits each day, you'll condition yourself to turn off the Type A traits that trigger negative stress reactions. Brain conditioning isn't spontaneous, so it might take a few weeks before you notice any difference in how you think and how you feel. A good way to see how you're progressing is to set a plan to paper. The following is a behavior modification action chart that you can use to gauge your success. Write down the Type A behaviors you think are causing the most stress symptoms, your plan of action for eliminating them, and the results. Seeing a concrete action plan on paper is a much better way of solving problems than just thinking about them.

Type A Behavior	Stress Symptoms	Action	Result of Action
Rushing to work	Headache; muscle tension	Get up earlier; do things the night before	Fewer headaches; less muscle tension
Multitasking	Stomach cramps; muscle pain	Prioritize tasks; delegate	Feel more relaxed
Worrying about everything	Nervousness; pacing back and forth	Take more breaks; do daily relaxation exercises	Feel more relaxed and less pressured
Doing everything myself	Anger; clenching jaw	Involve others; eliminate paperwork	Less angry; happier

The Stress-Sex Connection

Sex is a great way to relieve stress. Benefits include release of hormones that elevate mood, and exercise, which is a good stress reliever. But stress can also keep us from getting in the mood and not being able to perform sexually. Here's a common scenario:

You've had a bad day at the office and you come home still stressed out over an argument you had with your boss. When you try to have sex, your mind's not there and you can't get an erection. Without realizing that the problem is nothing more than stress, you force yourself into performing. It doesn't work. The next time you have sex, you remember what happened, which only makes you fail again. The harder you try, the worse it is and the stronger your conditioning becomes. Soon, performance anxiety is ingrained causing erectile dysfunction whenever you think about sex, which is the main reason men avoid sexual intimacy altogether.

Both men and women produce the sex hormones of FSH, LH, testosterone, and estrogen, although in different amounts. Chronic stress affects the concentration of all sex hormones because the body produces stress hormones such as cortisol at the expense of sex hormones like testosterone. In order to fight stress, our body shuts down sex mechanisms so that we're better able to deal with the more urgent and immediate needs of fight or flight. This change, called the stress-shift in hormone production, helps us respond to life-threatening situations by focusing hormone production for survival rather than procreation. The shift in hormones not only lowers sex drive but it can interfere with ovulation, sperm count, and fertility (see Figure 4.2).

For millions of men, erectile dysfunction is nothing more than a stress response that triggers a classic mind-body phenomenon. Sexual activity is under the control of the autonomic nervous system—we have no conscious control over it. When a man is aroused, nerve impulses cause blood vessels in the penis to dilate, allowing a flow of blood into the spongy tissue. At the same time, a circular muscle called a sphincter constricts to prevent blood from flowing back. During stress, blood vessels don't dilate fully and the sphincter fails to constrict, both contributing to erectile dysfunction. Negative events create a stress response that intensifies the more ingrained it becomes. And because physiological actions such as erection are controlled by the autonomic nervous system, the conditioning process is much harder to break.

As with any stress response, a variety of hormones are disrupted as well. Endorphins that block pain during stress also block LHRH (luteinizing hormone releasing hormone), which causes a drop in LH (luteinizing hormone), a hormone important in testosterone production. FSH, which stimulates sperm formation, also declines. To make things worse, cortisol, the main stress hormone, makes the testes less responsive to LH. The underlying power behind these reactions is the mind. Conditioning the brain is the key element in reversing it.

In many cases, simply recognizing stress as a contributing factor in or the cause of sexual problems is enough to bring about recovery. Ignoring the problem and not taking steps to address it can lead to anger, emotional disorders, depression, physical illness, and permanent loss of intimacy.

Figure 4.2: Sex Hormone Pathway (dashed lines represent inhibition)

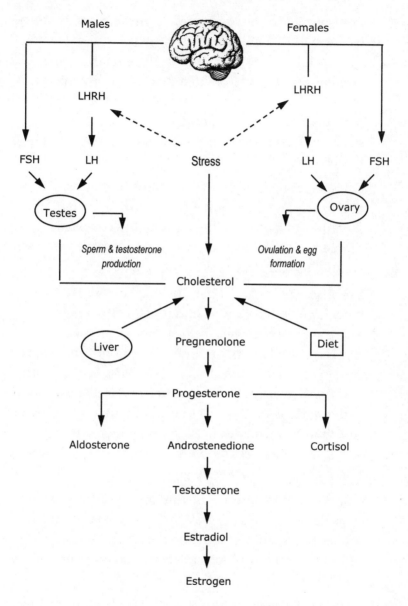

The following mind-body suggestions can help recondition the brain and reverse the process before it gets out of control.

- **Communicate your fears and desires.** Sexual problems will lead to loneliness and hostility if you don't share your feelings with your partner. Since many sexual problems start in the brain, and are typically the result of stress or anxiety, any treatment has to begin with both partners together. Simply sharing the anxiety, stress, and depression with someone is often enough for recovery.

- **Use special techniques to help eliminate sexual problems.** There are numerous resources, including therapy, available to address the causes of sexual problems. If you can't solve your problem on your own, counselors and clinicians are often able to help.

- **Exercise regularly.** People who exercise on a regular basis have better stamina and much better sex lives. There are three reasons for this. Firstly, physical exercise stimulates the release of hormones and triggers physiological reactions that boost libido. Secondly, the emotional awareness of being healthy and fit gives one a better outlook on life and translates into a better sex life. And thirdly, regular exercise stimulates growth of blood vessels and increases blood flow, which naturally leads to enhanced blood flow to genital areas.

- **Use stress relievers.** Use meditation, breathing exercises, yoga, laughter, and progressive muscle relaxation to reduce stress and tension. You'll be surprised at what just ten minutes a day of relaxation will do for your mindset and libido.

- **Get enough sleep.** Sleep is critical for health. It's also important for a good sex life because it reduces stress and keeps the immune system healthy. If you can't get your normal seven to eight hours a night, try power napping and see what that does for your energy and your sex drive.

- **Set the mood.** Getting in the mood for sex is not as easy as turning on a light switch. The best mood setter is communication with a partner, but some others are soothing music, aromas from scented candles that stimulate the senses, lighting that provides a romantic atmosphere, and massage, which triggers the relaxation response and induces emotional well-being. Using the bedroom for nothing but sleep and sex can also help let your libido know that when you're in that room it is for one of those purposes.

- **If all else fails, consult a physician.** Don't let embarrassment keep you from discussing with your physician any problems you may be experiencing sexually. Certain medications and medical conditions can affect sexual functioning. Ask your doctor about the sexual side effects of any new medications you may be taking.

Although an imbalance between sex and stress hormones can play a role in causing sexual problems, a major factor is negative conditioning created by stress itself. The most common sexual problems include unsatisfactory erections, untimely ejaculation, pain, and low libido. And sexual problems are very often the first sign of underlying serious medical issues. In women, for example, dulled desire may signal thyroid dysfunction or other hormonal troubles, and painful sex can even be an early symptom of pelvic cancer. And erectile dysfunction is now recognized as a possible early sign of impending cardiovascular disease.

Stress, Exercise, and Disease Prevention

Exercise is one of the best ways to relieve tension, make us feel more energized, help us sleep better (which by itself relieves stress), and give us a sense of well-being because it triggers the release of endorphins. But regular exercise also keeps the immune system healthy by decreasing the levels of cortisol and helping to stabilize insulin, both of which have negative effects on organ systems if too much is released. There's little doubt that regular exercise makes us more resistant to disease and infection and helps us recover from injuries more quickly.

An additional benefit of exercise is that in some cases it can be as effective in combating depression as prescription antidepressants. For example, in a study of 156 patients at Duke University, it was shown that those who walked briskly for thirty minutes at least three times a week were just as likely to recover from depression and have fewer relapses as those who were using antidepressants.[15] But exercise only helps as a stress reliever and in preventing disease if it's not stressful itself. Too many people force themselves to exercise or do exercises they don't enjoy doing. For me, jogging is too boring and more stressful than sitting in traffic. I'd rather take a brisk walk, lift weights, or watch television while on a treadmill for thirty minutes. If I get bored doing that, I'll go play golf (without a cart) or find something new to do.

The idea is to find a routine you enjoy and can stick with, not one you feel compelled to do because it's good for you. Pushing yourself too hard defeats the purpose. It makes it easier to quit and can actually have a negative effect on your health because it triggers the release of stress hormones. But the benefits of doing something as simple as walking three times a week for a total of sixty minutes will not only do wonders for you emotionally, it will significantly improve your odds of preventing disease in the first place or beating disease to which you succumb.

We're only now beginning to fully appreciate the correlation between the mind and immunity. At a recent NIH conference, paper after paper was presented showing the link between mind and body and between mind and a person's ability to fight off disease. More scientists than ever are recognizing the power one has to heal the body through mind control.

When it comes to stress, how do we know that it's actually the stress and not something else that's causing so many of our health problems? The evidence here is also mounting. In many parts of the world, where stress is not a normal part of life, coronary heart disease is rare. Once these people are exposed to the stresses of modern society, they become as susceptible as everyone else. Other studies also show conclusively that cholesterol levels, hypertension, diabetes, and other illnesses increase with stress. In one study of nine-to sixteen-year-olds, researchers found that even the routine act of reading out loud in front of classmates caused significant elevations in blood pressure.

Until recently, most illnesses were attributed to diet, heredity, lifestyle, and environment. Evidence now points to stress and the mind-body connection as a major factor in a wide range of illnesses from headaches to cancer. Many of these illnesses can be prevented or controlled by learning to use techniques and behavioral changes that trigger the healing power of the mind-body connection. Without a doubt, managing the stress in our lives is one of the single most important elements in ensuring that our immune system is ready when we need it most.

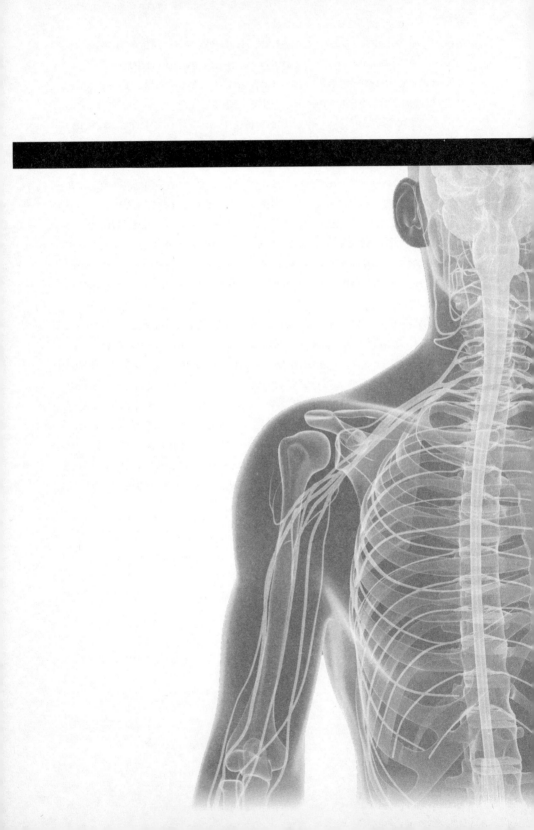

CHAPTER FIVE

Stress, Mental Health, and the Mind-Body Connection

Stress and Depression

As we have seen, stress is implicated in many cases of physical illness. So, given the mind-body connection, it will come as no surprise to learn that stress has an influence on our mental health, as well. The most widespread mental illness is depression, so much so that it's been called "the common cold" of mental illness. But as with the actual common cold, there are things we can do to mitigate depression as well, starting with changing the way we deal with stress. Of course, stress is not the only factor that contributes to depression; there are several. In some cases, a single cause is at the root of this problem; but in many cases a combination of factors is responsible. Genetics and family history, personality, medications, illnesses a person may have experienced, and life events such as death of a loved one or marital problems are all potential contributing factors.

Depression is often the result of a traumatic event or may be triggered by emotional stress. In these cases, psychologists treat the root cause by using individual coping strategies and stress management techniques. Stress-related depression can be overcome by increasing social interaction, communication, and involvement in activities. In fact, an ongoing network of social and moral support can help a person avoid developing mental health problems.

When researchers looked at specific examples of mental disorders, they discovered that stressful life events accounted for a large number of depression cases. One team of investigators looked at the life events of 185 depressed patients prior to the onset of their depression and found that in almost all cases there was an overwhelming excess of negative life events or events involving some sort of personal loss. When the stress effects of the 1979 Three Mile Island nuclear disaster in Pennsylvania were examined, researchers found that residents in close proximity to the disaster exhibited more stress symptoms and reported more depression, anxiety, and alienation than residents living in outlying areas, even eighteen months after the accident.[16] Similar studies have clearly shown that not only do depressed individuals experience more stressful life events in the months that precede the start of their depression, but that the risk of depression can increase six-fold during the six months following a tragic or intensely stressful episode.

Events especially likely to cause depression are the loss of relatives or loved ones, loss of a job, relocation, severely threatening episodes, and chronically undesirable experiences. However, in many cases, the stress events that cause depression are small, repetitive occurrences rather than major stress events. The cumulative effect of these "microstressors" can be as potent as "macrostressors" (if not more potent) because of the effects frequency and repetition have on conditioning and habit forming.

Regardless of its cause, depression can make us repeat our symptoms over and over, leaving us open to negative conditioning and habit formation. Unless we put into practice coping strategies to deal with depression, it will only get worse and more difficult to reverse. The good news is that depression is easy to recognize. Its signs and symptoms are a warning signal that allow us to deal with our stress immediately and effectively before we slip into a more chronic and dangerous state.

Signs and Symptoms of Depression

According to the standard medical definition, depression is a syndrome that may involve mood variations, insomnia, weight loss, guilt, and lack of reactivity to one's environment. We all experience these signs and symptoms at one time or another and we all exhibit them in different ways. Our depression can be something as simple as sadness over a loss or as severe as deep withdrawal in which we isolate ourselves and find it impossible to function normally.

During the last few decades, the rate of depression, and even the rate of suicide, has grown at an alarming rate. Sociologists attribute this to the mounting pressures and stresses of society. Individuals who commit or contemplate suicide are more likely to have experienced some traumatic life event, are more prone to depression, and have feelings of hopelessness and futility in dealing with life situations. On the other hand, those who seek professional help or learn to cope with stress are far less likely to think about suicide.

Depression that goes on for weeks or months is termed clinical, which is far more than the ordinary down moods everyone experiences now and then and that often pass after a day or two or a visit with a friend or a good movie. Clinical depression is a whole body disorder affecting the way we think and feel both physically and emotionally. It should always be taken seriously, since it can deepen and lead to thoughts of suicide or to violent behavior. The good news is that nearly 80 percent of people with clinical depression are treated successfully with medications, psychotherapy, or a combination of both. Even the most serious cases usually respond to the right therapy.

There are two types of severe depression: Major Depression and Bipolar Disorder (Manic-Depressive Illness). Individuals suffering with Major Depression find it almost impossible to carry on usual activities, to sleep, eat, or enjoy life. They derive no pleasure from anything they do and often sink deeper and deeper into despair. Although it can be a once in a lifetime occurrence, for many people it recurs several times over a lifespan. Because Major Depression can lead to more serious problems, and even suicide, professional treatment is critical. The most common symptoms are:

- Persistent sadness and/or feelings of emptiness
- Decreased energy levels; becoming fatigued more often
- Loss of interest or pleasure in day-to-day activities
- Decreased interest in intimacy and sex
- Sleep problems (insomnia, oversleeping, early-morning waking)
- Difficulty concentrating, remembering, or making decisions
- Feelings of hopelessness or pessimism
- Feelings of guilt, worthlessness, or helplessness
- Loss of appetite or weight; weight gain
- Thoughts of death or suicide or attempts at suicide
- Increased anger, moodiness, or irritability
- Excessive crying, sometimes for no apparent reason
- Recurring aches and pains that don't respond to treatment

Bipolar Disorder is characterized by severe mood swings, from extreme "highs" or mania, in which the person experiences elation and unbounded energy, to excessive "lows," in which he or she falls into a state of complete despair. Bipolar Disorder usually starts when people are in their early twenties and requires ongoing medical treatment. The most common symptoms of the manic phase are:

- Excessively "high" mood or euphoria
- Unexplained hostility or irritability
- Decreased need for sleep; waking up frequently
- Increased or excessive energy
- Increased talking and/or moving
- Increased frequency of sexual activity
- Racing thoughts
- Inability to make decisions or to concentrate
- Being easily distracted; inability to focus

Anyone experiencing four or more of these symptoms for more than two weeks needs to consult a physician or mental health specialist. While some people have a single episode of depression and never have another, or remain symptom-free for years, others have more frequent bouts or experience depression that may go on for months or years. Some people find that depression becomes more frequent as they get older, or that episodes only appear at certain times or during certain activities. Whatever the reason, if depression becomes more frequent or begins to last longer each time, it needs to be addressed before symptoms get more serious and out of hand.

Often people have other illness along with depression. Sometimes another illness comes first; but other times the depression comes first. One of the worst mistakes people can make is ignoring the other illness and not getting treated for both. Some of the most common disorders that occur along with depression are anxiety disorders, obsessive-compulsive behavior, panic disorder, social phobia, addiction, heart disease, cancer, HIV/AIDS, diabetes, and Parkinson's disease. Studies have found that treating depression can help in treating these other illnesses.

Depression Rating Quiz

Depression can be nothing more than feeling down about what happened on a particular day or as serious as having thoughts of suicide. The following quiz is designed to help determine whether someone is just having a bad few days or is suffering from clinical depression.

1. Have you lost complete interest in things you used to enjoy?   Yes ☐   No ☐

2. Do you find yourself feeling sad or blue every day?   Yes ☐   No ☐

3. Are you lethargic or restless and unable to sit still?   Yes ☐   No ☐

4. Do you have feelings of guilt or worthlessness?   Yes ☐   No ☐

5. Has there been an increase or decrease in your appetite or weight?   Yes ☐   No ☐

6. Do you have thoughts of death or suicide?   Yes ☐   No ☐

7. Do you have trouble concentrating or remembering?   Yes ☐   No ☐

8. Do you have insomnia or do you sleep too much?   Yes ☐   No ☐

9. Are you tired all of the time?   Yes ☐   No ☐

10. Do you find yourself worrying much of the time?   Yes ☐   No ☐

11. Do you experience feelings of pessimism or hopelessness?   Yes ☐   No ☐

12. Are you experiencing more sexual problems than you used to?　　Yes ☐　No ☐

13. Have you started drinking more often?　　Yes ☐　No ☐

14. Are you experiencing unexplained pains or aches?　　Yes ☐　No ☐

15. Are you experiencing digestive problems more often?　　Yes ☐　No ☐

You are suffering from depression if you answered YES to either question 1 or 2. If you answered YES to at least three of the next seven questions (3–9), chances are you're suffering from depression. If you answered YES to questions 10–15, it may also be the result of depression. So what do you do? Psychiatrists recommend one or a combination of therapies:

1. **Seek treatment, perhaps with antidepressant medication.** Antidepressants are not addictive or habit forming. They work in cases of severe depression by balancing chemicals in the brain, and may be useful in people with mild to moderate depression. Typically, it takes up to two to four weeks for patients to begin feeling the effects.

2. **Undergo psychotherapy.** The most common types are behavioral therapy that focuses on current behaviors, cognitive therapy that focuses on thoughts and beliefs, and interpersonal therapy that focuses on current relationships. Psychotherapy is basically "talk-therapy" that helps patients change negative styles of thinking and behaving or helps them understand and work through troubled personal relationships that may cause depression or make it worse.

Nutrition, Stress, and Depression

Diet therapy to treat depression was first used in the 1950s when it was discovered that a variety of nutrients are necessary to maintain proper brain chemistry. The more psychiatrists looked, the more they found that many of their depressed patients had poor eating habits. More recent studies have shown that people who are sad more often than normal have low levels of folic acid, and that those who don't get enough of it are less likely to benefit from mood-elevating drugs like Prozac.

So the expression "you are what you eat" became popular because we discovered that there really *is* a link between the things we eat and how we feel. In fact, psychologists now agree that people with some types of depression have certain things in common, two of which are diet and stress. They found that besides the usual physiological effects on the body, stress and anxiety prevent vitamin and mineral absorption and disrupt nutrient pathways that manufacture important brain chemicals like serotonin (5-HT), noradrenalin, melatonin, and tryptophan (See Figure 5.1).

Serotonin, linked to mood and called the "stress immunizer," and noradrenalin, linked to nerve transmission and energy, are derived from amino acids founds in meats, dairy products, and other food supplements. When the levels of these chemicals decrease, normal brain and bodily functions are impaired. Low levels of serotonin can lead to severe depression, insomnia, and suicidal behavior, and researchers found that patients with the lowest serotonin levels tend to exhibit the most aggressive or violent behavior. Medications that boost serotonin work because they reduce negative stress reactions.

Figure 5.1: Pathway Through Which Dietary Protein Is Converted to Brain Chemicals

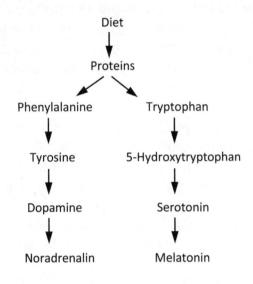

The amino acid tryptophan is converted to serotonin in the brain and eventually to melatonin, a hormone important in establishing and maintaining biological rhythms. Like serotonin, low levels of melatonin have been associated with depression, premenstrual syndrome, addiction, decreased immunity, and aging. The relationship between stress, depression, and serotonin is important because one of the vital functions of serotonin is to induce drowsiness and sleep. Sleep, in turn, is an effective mechanism for helping us relax and relieve symptoms of depression. Other than being a precursor for serotonin, researchers have found that tryptophan may increase pain tolerance, relieve premenstrual symptoms, control appetite, fight nicotine addiction, soothe anxiety, and induce sleep.

Researchers have also shown that low levels of the neurotransmitter noradrenalin may cause depression. Eating foods rich in the amino acid phenylalanine, which is converted to tyrosine, the building block of noradrenalin, can help us fight off the onset of stress-related depression. As we continue to learn more about nutrition and its effects on disease and mental health, we're discovering that food can trigger changes in virtually every part of our body.

Foods that help stimulate production of brain serotonin include: whole grains, barley, brown rice, carrots, celery, corn, oatmeal, onions, potatoes, radishes, squash, turnips, and yams. Turkey is also good because it contains the amino acid tryptophan, which is converted to serotonin. But since proteins compete with carbohydrates for entry into the brain, you should alternate a high protein meal with a high carbohydrate meal. The best way to elevate serotonin levels, however, is to moderate protein intake and eat a large variety of complex carbohydrates, especially whole grains, fruits, and vegetables.

Becoming Depression Resistant

Perhaps the single most important factor that separates a depression-prone from a depression-resistant person is the ability to cope effectively with negative life stress. For example, when patients at a community mental health center participated in a thirty-hour program designed to teach relaxation exercises, social skills, and attitude and behavior modification, they had significantly lower levels of depression and more ability to solve problems and control their lives than individuals who didn't participate.

This was even more apparent in different ethnic groups. Researchers who looked at the mental health records of various ethnic groups found that when an ethnic group formed a large community and, thus, a substantial social support network, hospitalization rates due to mental health problems were very low. They also found that when an ethnic group began to constitute a small minority of a neighborhood, the rates of mental illness and hospitalization increased dramatically because they no longer had a buffer against the stressful life events they weren't able to deal with alone.

Unless a depression is severe and caused by a medical/physical condition or deep emotional problems, certain coping strategies can be used to reverse or lessen depression. Here are the eight coping techniques found to be the most effective in treating stress-related depression:

1. **Spend more time with family and friends.** Seeing family and friends on a regular basis does wonders for mental health. Schedule get-togethers, have game nights, and entertain more often, because stress and depression seem to decrease as interactions increase.

2. **Train yourself to think positively.** Often, having a negative attitude is a habit we acquire over a lifetime. The more we focus on the negative, the more conditioned we become to develop a negative personality that is more prone to depression. We can literally train ourselves to think positively and become happier by simply focusing on the positive aspects of our lives. Every day, think of something positive in your life and be grateful for it. Remind yourself how lucky you are for the things that make your life worth living.

3. **Exercise.** Walking, running, or getting up and going to the gym will stimulate both your nervous and immune systems and give you a sense of well-being. In addition, just the act of doing something to improve yourself will have a positive effect on your mental attitude.

4. **Work on your communication skills.** One of the main sources of stress between family members is a lack of communication. Talking with each other improves relationships, and stress is much easier to handle when it's not left to fester. Some ways to express feelings in a constructive and positive way are:

   • **Don't dwell on the negative.** Try to not be critical. Always make communication a mutual dialogue, not a monologue or lecture.

- **Write letters.** Letter writing can be an effective method of expression if you're having trouble communicating verbally. Writing feelings down on paper makes them easier to discuss because you have them right there in front of you.

- **Learn to really listen.** Listening is important because it shows that you're interested in what the other person is saying. Make eye contact to show that you're paying attention. Don't respond too quickly. And always give the other person a chance to finish what he or she is trying to say.

- **Avoid non-pertinent issues.** Don't bring up past grievances or troubles you've had, even if they deal indirectly with the present discussion. If you know that certain issues are going to cause anger and resentment, don't bring them up deliberately or in a negative way.

- **Focus on the underlying issue causing the problem.** Talk about one thing at a time. Keeping to one topic prevents other issues from complicating the picture and making communication more difficult.

5. **Eat a well-balanced, low fat diet.** Research has shown that fattening foods can affect a variety of biochemical reactions that affect mood. Furthermore, eating foods that contribute to the production of serotonin and melatonin may actually help balance brain chemicals and prevent depression. Losing some weight in the process just adds to the positive feelings you'll have about yourself.

6. **Try some lemon balm extract.** A few drops in a glass of water can have a calming effect. Because it's all natural, you can take it up to three times a day whenever you're stressed and need to calm down quickly.

7. **Develop social support systems.** Social support groups like friends, church community, and family can brighten your outlook on life and help lessen depression and anxiety. Social support networks are recommended by psychiatrists and psychologists as a tool to help treat mental health problems because they have proven to be one of the best methods for enhancing relationships, communication, and interactions.

8. **Become more involved.** Sometimes all it takes to get your mind off your problems is getting involved in activities, social gatherings, civic organizations, or anything else that will give you a sense of worth and accomplishment. Many individuals who are depressed because of loneliness find that involvement alone is the answer to their depression.

Coping strategies for stress-related depression also include relaxation exercises that I will describe at length in later chapters. But, as with any health problem, the best treatment depends on the personality type and character of the individual and the extent of depression. Learning to recognize the early signs and symptoms of depression and then using coping strategies to deal with it as soon as possible is the best way to bring about a healthy and lasting recovery.

Anxiety and Related Disorders

After depression, anxiety disorders are the most common mental health problem. Rather than a single illness, anxiety disorders are grouped into the following:

Panic Disorder: Repeated episodes of intense fear that strike often and without warning. Physical symptoms include chest pain, heart palpitations, shortness of breath, dizziness, abdominal distress, feelings of unreality, and fear of dying.

Obsessive-Compulsive Disorder (OCD): Repeated, unwanted thoughts or compulsive behaviors that seem impossible to stop or control.

Post-Traumatic Stress Disorder (PTSD): Persistent symptoms that occur after experiencing a traumatic event such as rape or other criminal assault, war, child abuse, natural disasters, or crashes. Nightmares, flashbacks, numbing of emotions, depression, and feeling angry, irritable, or distracted and being easily startled are common.

Phobias: Two major types of fears are social phobia and specific phobia. People with social phobia have an overwhelming and disabling fear of scrutiny, embarrassment, or humiliation in social situations, which leads to avoidance of many potentially pleasurable and meaningful activities. People with specific phobia experience extreme, disabling, and irrational fear of something that poses little or no actual danger. The fear leads to avoidance of objects or situations and can cause people to limit their lives unnecessarily.

Generalized Anxiety Disorder (GAD): Constant, exaggerated worrisome thoughts and tension about everyday routine life events and activities, lasting at least six months. Almost always anticipating the worst even though there is little reason to expect it; accompanied by physical symptoms, such as fatigue, trembling, muscle tension, headache, or nausea.

Treatments for anxiety disorders are often a combination of medication and specific types of psychotherapy. More medications are available than ever before and include both antidepressants and benzodiazepines. Two clinically proven and effective forms of psychotherapy are behavioral therapy and cognitive-behavioral therapy. Behavioral therapy focuses on changing specific actions and uses several techniques to stop unwanted behaviors. Cognitive-behavioral therapy teaches patients to understand and change their thinking patterns so they can react differently to the situations that cause them anxiety.

Many people with anxiety disorders benefit from joining a self-help or support group and sharing their problems and concerns with others. Talking with a trusted friend or member of the clergy can also provide support, but it's not a substitute for care from a mental health professional. Stress management techniques and meditation can help people with anxiety disorders calm themselves and can often enhance the effects of therapy. Aerobic exercise may also have a calming effect. Since caffeine, certain illicit drugs, and even some over-the-counter cold medications can aggravate the symptoms of anxiety disorders, they should be avoided. Check with your physician or pharmacist before taking any additional medications.

It is common for an anxiety disorder to accompany depression, eating disorders, substance abuse or another anxiety disorder. Anxiety disorders can also coexist with physical disorders. In such instances, the accompanying disorders will also need to be treated. However, before beginning any treatment, it's important to have a thorough medical examination to rule out other possible causes of symptoms.

Loneliness Is a State of Mind

Despite the fact that we sometimes need to be by ourselves, as humans we're basically social creatures. We feed off each another, enjoy the interaction of friends, and need relationships in order to maintain emotional well-being. A growing number of studies show that the healthiest among us are married, have intimate relationships, or are involved in activities in which we interact with other people.

But at times the mind perceives loneliness even when we're not alone. How often have we been in a crowded room or surrounded by people, even people we know, and still felt alone? In those cases, loneliness can be as much a state of mind as it is a condition. When we become accustomed to thinking of ourselves as being alone it can become habit forming, leading to depression and other health problems. Eventually loneliness becomes a self-fulfilling prophecy. According to experts, the key to overcoming loneliness is to reach out to others instead of waiting for others to reach out to you. The biggest mistake we make is assuming that someone will recognize our loneliness and help us do something about it. So here are some ways to overcome the tendency to pull away and become that lonely person:

- **Expand your circle of friends.** Don't feel sorry for yourself and dwell on how lonely you're feeling or how few friends you have. You'll never expand your circle of friends or break the cycle of loneliness by avoiding people. It's a two-way street in that you shouldn't expect much if you're not willing to do something about it yourself.

- **Volunteer.** The fastest way to get your mind off the fact that you're lonely is to reach out and help others. Serving others is not only a noble thing to do, it gives you a sense of worth and accomplishment and makes you realize how truly blessed you are.

- **Learn to enjoy your introverted side.** Although as human beings we're social by nature, it's important that you enjoy your own company at times and that you're comfortable being alone. By discovering things you like to do by yourself, you won't feel the need to be around others in order to keep from being lonely.

- **Get involved in a mutual aid, self-help support group.** If our loneliness is caused by a physical or emotional problem, people who are experiencing similar problems can help us get through them. In fact, there's a strong correlation between the amount of social support and our physical and mental health.

Good mental health is often linked to a healthy mind-body connection. And based on clinical studies, the one coping strategy that stands out more than any other in helping overcome emotional problems is the use of social support networks and becoming involved with other people. No other stress therapy has had so much impact on so many different disorders, including depression and anxiety.

As social animals, we need to relate to and communicate with others. Without this human component, most of us would be unable to deal with the mounting stresses that we're subjected to at work and at home. The seventeenth century poet, John Donne, recognized this strong human need in these lines from his famous poem:

No man is an island entire of itself;

every man is a piece of the continent, a part of the main;

if a clod be washed away by the sea,

Europe is the less

as well as if a promontory were,

as well as any manner of thy friends or of thine own were;

any man's death diminishes me, for I am involved in mankind.

And therefore, never send to know for whom the bell tolls;

it tolls for thee.

Unless we participate in relationships with other people, we'll continue to have high rates of stress-induced disease, mental health problems, and suicide. In a society that's becoming increasingly complex and creates more and more stress, we all have a stake in each other's lives, our health, and our well-being.

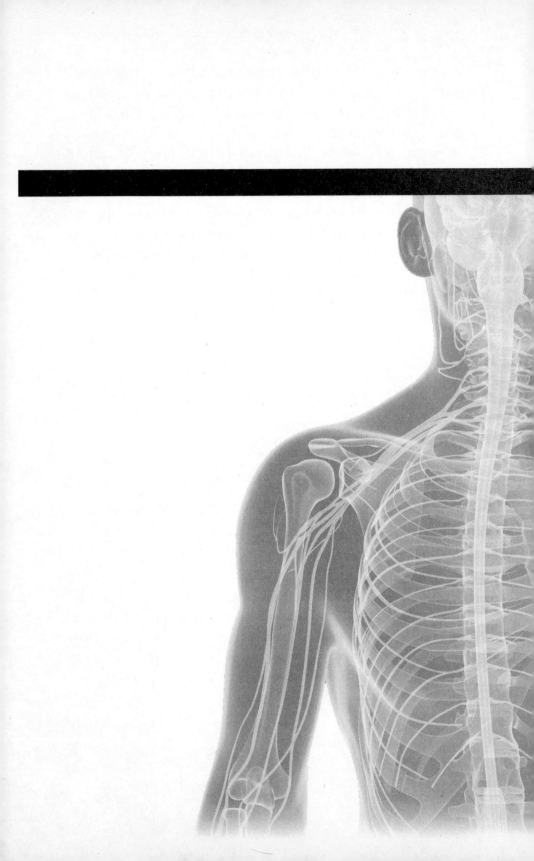

CHAPTER SIX

Aging and the Mind-Body Connection

Aging: Everybody's Doing It

The current proportion of older adults in the United States is unprecedented in our nation's history, with the number of Americans aged sixty-five or older predicted to reach almost ninety million by 2050. This rapid aging of the population is being driven by the birth of the post-World War II generation known as Baby Boomers, and increasingly longer life spans due to medical advances that keep us healthy well into our eighties. But while an aging population means that we are extending lifespan, it also means that our minds and our bodies will need to stay healthy in order for us to maintain a good quality of life during those extended years.

As we age, our cells and our organ systems begin to deteriorate more rapidly. Healing and recovery come more slowly as muscle and nerve function decline. Metabolism slows, blood vessels narrow, immune function decreases, our circulatory and respiratory systems are less efficient, and our ability to repair damaged DNA is much lower. Combined with poor nutrition, stress, and unhealthy lifestyles, these normal effects of aging also produce changes in our mind-body connection that make it more likely that we become even more susceptible to negative life events.

Many of the diseases that claimed our ancestors, like tuberculosis, diarrhea, enteritis, and syphilis are no longer the threats they once were. However, other diseases have continued to be leading causes of death every year since 1900. By 1910, heart disease became the leading cause of death. Since 1938, cancer has held the second position every year. Heart disease and cancer pose their greatest risks as people age, as do other chronic diseases and conditions, such as stroke, chronic respiratory diseases, Alzheimer's disease, and diabetes.

Because the aging mind-body connection is not as finely tuned as it once was, stress, which depresses immunity, makes the elderly more susceptible to a host of diseases. Together with the stress of aging, illness and disease intensify conditioned stress responses, which make the elderly even more prone to stress-related disorders. The more stress episodes the body has to respond to and overcome, the greater the damage will eventually be.

Scientists are getting close to pinpointing the complex mechanisms of aging and why some individuals, despite unhealthy habits and behaviors, are genetically programmed to live longer than others. But for now, we're certain that the process of aging alters the critical neuro-endocrine-immune system that is at the heart of the mind-body connection and is a key to keeping us healthy and disease-free. Doing everything we can to keep that system working ensures both physical and mental well-being.

Life Satisfaction Quiz: How Well Are You Aging?

Biological aging is the result of cell death and the gradual breakdown of organ systems. As we age, we allow negative perceptions of aging to shape our behavior and attitudes, which, together, cause negative conditioning. The result is psychological aging, which triggers severe stress reactions and makes us more susceptible to mental health problems as we get older. When these stress reactions get worse, physical symptoms crop up and intensify the stress reactions. This vicious cycle is often difficult to reverse and accelerates the aging process. Successful aging, then, really depends on how we perceive life in our golden years and how well we cope with the challenges that life throws at us as we age.

So how successful are you at aging compared to others your age? The following are some life statements about which older people feel differently. Read each statement and check whether you agree or disagree with it. A scoring key at the end of the list should give you an idea of how successful you are at aging well.

Life Statement	Agree	Disagree
These are the best years of my life.	☐	☐
As I get older, things are better than I thought.	☐	☐
I'm usually not bored because I find things to do.	☐	☐
Things are as interesting to me as they ever were.	☐	☐
I feel as energetic today as I did last year.	☐	☐
Most days I'm happy and satisfied.	☐	☐
I don't think that much about my age.	☐	☐
I visit family and friends on a regular basis.	☐	☐
Compared to others my age, I feel pretty lucky.	☐	☐
I look forward to the future.	☐	☐
When I think back, I'm content with what I've done.	☐	☐
I make plans for activities I'll do a month from now.	☐	☐

Life Statement

	Agree	Disagree
If I had to do it over, I wouldn't change most things.	☐	☐
I'm as happy today as I was when I was younger.	☐	☐
I've provided well for my retirement.	☐	☐
Compared to others my age, I'm healthy and fit.	☐	☐
I've accomplished most of what I wanted to do.	☐	☐
Despite what's in the news, I believe things are good.	☐	☐
I'm usually not lonely.	☐	☐
Compared to others my age, I have an active life.	☐	☐
I try to exercise thirty minutes at least four times a week.	☐	☐
I get at least six to seven hours of sleep on most nights.	☐	☐
I feel free to do most things I want.	☐	☐
I don't use tobacco products.	☐	☐
I drink no more than two glasses of wine or beer a day.	☐	☐
I feel less stress now than I did when I was younger.	☐	☐
Compared to others my age, I still enjoy sex.	☐	☐
I eat at least five servings of fruits and vegetables a day.	☐	☐
When shopping, I make it a habit to look at labels.	☐	☐
I have an annual physical, including blood work.	☐	☐

Scoring key: One point for each statement you agree with.
25–30: High Life Satisfaction. You're aging better than most people your age because you don't let your age get in the way of your enjoying life. You have positive attitudes and a good outlook that keeps you young at heart. This bodes well for your mind and your body.

14–24: Average Life Satisfaction. Your attitude may be keeping you from being fully satisfied with your life. Participating in more physical and mental activities, widening your circle of friends, and taking up a hobby or two will improve your outlook. Don't allow negative attitudes and behaviors to ruin your golden years.

0–14: Low Life Satisfaction. You're not aging successfully. You need to take charge of your life by getting out and meeting people, joining clubs, doing volunteer work, eating right, and exercising more. Your low score may also be an indication of depression, which can lead to more serious issues. One of the best ways to reverse a negative attitude is to become involved with a social network of people your age.

Human Lifespan: Is There an Age Limit?

Jeanne Louise Calment of France, who died in 1997 at the age of 122, has the longest confirmed lifespan on record. Previously, Shigechiyo Izumi of Japan held the record as the oldest living person until he died of pneumonia in 1986 at the ripe old age of 120. Also from Japan, Jiroemon Kimura died in 2013 at 116 years old. What was their secret? And are we all capable of living that long? The answers, according to experts on aging, lie in our genes, our environment, and our lifestyle. But a more interesting question is: If Shigechiyo Izumi did not get pneumonia or any other disease, how much longer could he have lived? In other words, what is a human being's maximum lifespan?

The latest research on genes and how they affect aging seems to suggest that the maximum lifespan is indeed about 120 years. The difference between human lifespan and that of other species lies in our twenty-three pairs of chromosomes, the pieces of DNA that make up everything about us. In yeast, for example, fourteen known genes are related to aging. In fruit flies and worms, genes have been isolated that have a direct effect on their lifespan. Scientists have even manipulated the genes of various species to extend their lifespans, some by as much as twice the normal length.

A few decades ago, scientists learned that the 100 trillion or so cells in the human body, which continually divide and multiply, have a finite lifespan. Once a certain number of cell divisions take place, the DNA can no longer duplicate. This is what we know as senescence. Each cell has tails on each end called telomeres, which get shorter with each cell division. When DNA loses a certain number of telomeres, it signals the cell that it can no longer divide.

Despite human lifespan being programmed by genes and the architecture of DNA, each one of us can maximize lifespan by paying attention to the other two factors: environment and lifestyle. Based on the latest census data, centenarians are on the rise and more are staying active and healthy. By using the strategies in this chapter to keep the mind-body connection working like it did when we were younger, there's no reason we, too, can't live to one hundred and beyond.

Stress Hormones During Aging

As we age, stress hormones begin to affect our bodies in different ways and make the stress response even more acute and much more damaging. They can actually speed up the normal aging processes by depressing immune function and accelerating cell death. Stress hormones can also affect the way in which the brain and the central nervous system operate and interact. Studies done at Wake Forest University School of Medicine, for example, suggest that stress hormones may be responsible for some of the structural changes taking place within the aging brain.[17] Other studies have found that hormones released as a result of stress decrease brain function during aging and lead to dramatic changes in how the mind-body connection responds to life events.

So what is it about stress hormones that cause such profound changes to the aging process? The answer, according to scientists, may lie in the hippocampus, the same area of the brain involved in learning and memory. It turns out that another important function of the hippocampus is regulation of cortisol, the stress hormone most responsible for negative health effects. The chain of events that occur during stress reactions seem to play a vital role in immune system breakdown and premature aging.

- Stress causes the pituitary gland to produce ACTH, which then stimulates the adrenal glands to release cortisol.

- Cortisol increases the risk of diabetes and osteoporosis, causes a breakdown in immune function, and damages the hippocampus.

- Damage to the hippocampus makes the body release even more cortisol.

- Excess cortisol further depresses the immune system and damages the hippocampus, which makes one even more susceptible to illness and disease.

The other hormone that wreaks havoc on aging systems, and actually accelerates the aging process, is insulin. Insulin spikes, caused by eating too many carbohydrates or high glycemic foods, cause the body to release more cortisol in an effort to balance glucose levels. The end result is even more cortisol, depressed immune function, and damage to cells and organ systems. To prevent this from happening, limit the amount of sugar you eat; exercise, which reduces insulin levels and makes cells more efficient at responding to insulin; and manage stress levels, one of the best ways to reduce cortisol in general.

Growth Hormone Cycles During Aging

Human growth hormone (HGH) stimulates growth, increases bone density, helps repair damaged tissue, increases metabolism, promotes muscle growth, and decreases body fat. It's highest at puberty and begins to decline by about 15 percent for every decade thereafter. By the time we're fifty-five, our HGH levels are six times lower than they were at age fifteen, which accounts for many of the physical effects we experience as we get older. This is bad news for both the mind and body since we're less able to use the mind-body connection to repair damaged cells and tissues. The good news is that we can stimulate our pituitary to release more HGH without resorting to HGH replacement therapy.

HGH has a predictable circadian rhythm. It remains fairly steady throughout the day, but rises slightly in the evening and then begins to surge one hour after the onset of sleep until it reaches a peak during the early morning hours (Figure 6.1). Knowing this pattern is helpful because we can do certain things to maximize HGH release.

Figure 6.1: Circadian Rhythm of Human Growth Hormone

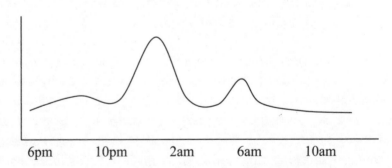

6pm 10pm 2am 6am 10am

One important fact we've learned in the past decade is that simple carbohydrates tend to switch off HGH secretion, and since most of our HGH is released at night while we sleep, the worst foods to eat before bed are empty sugary snacks. Carbs also cause a spike in our insulin levels, and insulin also decreases HGH levels. So to get our HGH levels up naturally, here are a few tips:

- **Eat protein and healthy fats before bed.** Greek yogurt is good, together with some nuts, low fat cheeses, peanut butter, or high fiber foods, which stabilize blood sugar levels and prevent insulin spikes. Avoid saturated fats and simple sugars.

- **Avoid fats one to two hours before you exercise.** This tends to decrease HGH levels. The best foods to eat before a workout are proteins and complex carbohydrates like whole-grain breads, starchy vegetables, and beans.

- **Perform compound versus isolation exercises.** Compound exercises like squats, deadlifts, bench presses, and overhead presses utilize multiple joints and are much more effective in stimulating HGH than bicep curls and dumbbell kickbacks.

- **Choose High Intensity Interval Training (HIIT) over long cardio sessions.** HIIT is extremely effective at boosting metabolism and stimulating an HGH response. For example, instead of getting on a treadmill and walking at a steady pace for an hour, try this: warm up for five minutes, then peddle as fast as you can for thirty seconds; slow down and peddle slowly for a minute and then peddle as fast as you can again for thirty seconds. Do this for six cycles and your metabolism will be revved up for the next forty-eight hours instead of the two hours it would be after a long cardio session.

- **Never exercise for more than an hour.** After about forty-five minutes to an hour of exercise, your body begins to release cortisol, which not only breaks down muscle but will cause your body to produce less HGH. So plan your exercise sessions wisely because, in this case, more is not necessarily better.

- **Take some glutamine at night before bed.** Glutamine is an amino acid that many bodybuilders take to help repair muscle tissue after a workout. It also happens to increase HGH when taken at night before bed.

- **Snack on goji berries.** Several clinical studies have shown that goji berries, which are rich in antioxidants like beta-carotene, naturally stimulate the release of HGH. Used for more than 5,000 years in Asia, goji berries also boost immunity, improve circulation, reduce blood sugar, fight tumor growth, and slow aging.

Sex Hormones and Aging

Men and women both produce testosterone and estrogen, though in different amounts. As we age, the levels of both hormones decline and with that decline comes anxiety, emotional upset, and physiological problems, all of which begin to affect the mind-body connection. In women, the decline of estrogen marks the beginning of menopause, while in men the decrease in testosterone causes increased fat storage, a breakdown in muscle, and depressed libido. But declining testosterone isn't exclusively a male problem. Because it's naturally made by the ovaries to help make estrogen, a sudden decrease in a woman's testosterone is also associated with depressed sex drive and reduced sexual behavior.

For older women, difficulty becoming aroused because of low testosterone levels often leads to an inability to reach orgasm. In these cases, testosterone therapy might prove effective. Studies have shown that women who use testosterone supplements or testosterone boosters have marked improvement in both sexual desire and sexual function. Some of these testosterone boosters are listed later in this section.

In the 1940s, medical experts had officially coined the medical term andropause, which is the male equivalent of menopause. It wasn't until the 1990s that the medical community began to look at this condition more seriously, and researchers began to link low testosterone levels with various diseases and behavioral problems. But unlike menopause, where estrogen levels drop suddenly, andropause doesn't mean a sudden drop in testosterone. The decrease is gradual, with men losing approximately 1 percent of their testosterone each year after the age of thirty. So by the time a man is sixty years old, he is producing 30 percent less than he did thirty years ago. This leads to increased risk of heart disease, osteoporosis, depression, erectile dysfunction, and fatigue, not to mention a lowered sex drive.

When the body no longer produces enough estrogen and testosterone, one of the most common remedies is hormone supplementation in the form of pills, gels, or shots. The downside to this approach is the risk of adverse side effects and the fact that the hormone supplements are interfering with the body's own hormone regulatory system. For example, testosterone replacement therapy in men can cause enlarged prostate, breast growth, fluid retention, increased cholesterol, kidney problems, hypertension, sleep apnea, and shrunken testicles due to the body's decreased production of its own testosterone. In fact, bodybuilders on steroids stop producing testosterone because the body senses that it is getting enough of it. The brain signals the testes to literally shut down.

Nutrition and the Aging Process

Research over the past decade has shown that common diseases associated with aging, such as heart disease, diabetes, and hypertension, can be prevented simply by controlling the foods we eat and the supplements we take. Together with exercise and a healthy lifestyle, nutrition is key to keeping the mind-body connection working well into old age.

So why is it that so many older individuals develop poor eating habits as they age? At ninety years of age, my mother, for example, would pour salt and sugar on everything, regardless of whether it was already salty or sweet. One reason is that older persons have fewer taste buds and smell receptors, so food tastes too bland to them unless it's highly seasoned. Unfortunately, many unhealthy foods are very highly seasoned and flavorful, which is attractive to those whose taste mechanism is not what it once was.

But another reason older people eat poorly is linked to— you guessed it: stress.

Older persons can become fearful, anxious, lonely, and depressed, all of which can lead to illness and emotional problems that cause poor eating habits. Weak gums and teeth add to the problem because many nutritious foods are not always easy to chew. Poor eating habits develop over time, altering levels of stress hormones, affecting the aging process, and leading to age-related illness and disease.

In order to keep the mind and the body as healthy as possible during the aging process, diet and nutrition are vital. In the words of Hippocrates, the father of medicine: "Let food be thy medicine, and let medicine be thy food." Healthy foods are a natural medicine that affects memory, keeps nerve, muscle, and bone cells healthy, and prevents illness and disease. Knowing which foods, supplements, and brain exercises enhance both physical and mental fitness will ensure successful aging. The following checklist is designed to identify the often overlooked warning signs of poor nutritional health. Read each statement, which has a nutritional risk value from 1 to 4. Add each "yes" answer and then total up your nutritional health score.

Nutritional Health Questions

	Yes	Points
I have an illness or condition that has made me change the kind and/or amount of food I eat.	☐	2
I eat fewer than two meals per day.	☐	3
I eat few fruits and vegetables or milk products.	☐	2
I have three or more drinks of alcohol every day.	☐	2
I have tooth or mouth problems that make it difficult for me to eat.	☐	2
I don't always have the money to buy the food I need.	☐	4
I eat alone most of the time.	☐	1
I take three or more different prescribed or over-the-counter drugs each day.	☐	1
Without wanting to, I have lost or gained ten pounds in the last six months.	☐	2
I am not always physically able to shop, cook, and/or feed myself.	☐	2
TOTAL		_____

Scoring key:

0–2: Excellent. Recheck your nutritional score in six months.

3–5: Moderate risk. See what you can do to improve your eating habits and lifestyle. Recheck your nutritional score in three months.

6 or more: High nutritional risk. Bring this checklist next time you see your doctor or other healthcare provider. Ask for help to improve your nutritional health.

Older people need to pay attention to nutritional warning labels because four out of five adults have chronic diseases that are directly affected by diet. Less than 15 percent of adults eat the minimum amount of fruits and vegetables. A third of older people live alone, which affects emotional well-being and eating habits. Older people typically take multiple drugs daily, which can cause side effects such as nausea, change in taste, and decreased appetite. And many older adults have trouble walking, shopping, and cooking food, all of which contributes to stress, poor eating habits, and, consequently, poor health.

Good nutrition is one of the cornerstones of maintaining a healthy mind-body connection during aging. Foods can boost immunity, increase brainpower, and keep us emotionally balanced. So no matter what your genetic makeup is, successful aging is possible only if you fuel your body with the nutrients that keep you both physically and mentally fit. Here are the guidelines that will promote health and reduce the risk of chronic diseases as you age.

- **Don't skip meals.** Skipping meals may cause your metabolism to slow down or lead you to eat more high-calorie, high-fat foods at your next meal or snack. Breakfast is especially important because studies have found that people who eat a good high-protein breakfast burn more calories throughout the day and are less hungry. It seems that the healthiest follow the rule: Eat breakfast like a king, lunch like a queen, and dinner like a pauper.

- **Eat high-fiber foods.** Whole grain breads, pasta, cereals, beans, fruits, and vegetables. Supplement with psyllium fiber (found in products like Metamucil) to help keep you regular, lower your cholesterol, and decrease your risk of heart disease and diabetes.

- **Choose lean meats.** Lean beef, turkey breast, fish, or baked chicken with the skin removed will lower the amount of fat and calories in your meals. As you age, metabolism decreases and your body needs fewer calories.

- **Have three servings of vitamin D-fortified foods every day.** Most of the population is deficient in vitamin

D, arguably the most important vitamin for lowering the risk of almost every disease. Low-fat milk, yogurt, and cheese are high in calcium, as well as vitamin D, which keeps bones strong as you age. An important fact that most women don't realize is that calcium is not absorbed very well without vitamin D, and this might lead to an increased risk of osteoporosis. To be sure that you're getting enough vitamin D, ask your doctor if you should be supplementing with at least 1000 mg.

- **Choose foods fortified with vitamin B12.** If you're over the age of fifty, you may have difficulty absorbing adequate amounts of B12, which then affects production of red blood cells and leaves you less energized. To make sure you have enough, eat fortified breakfast cereals and take a Vitamin B12 supplement.

- **Eat nutrition-rich snacks.** Keep nutrition-rich snacks like dried fruit, nuts, whole wheat crackers, peanut butter, and low-fat cheese on hand. Eat only small amounts of these foods because they are still high in calories. Avoid high-fat, high-salt, and high-sugar snacks like cake, candy, chips, and soda,

- **Drink plenty of water.** You may notice that you feel less thirsty as you get older, but your body still needs water to stay healthy and build muscle. Also, remember that drinks like coffee and tea are diuretics, so you'll be losing water if you drink too much of these.

It's easier to eat well when you plan for your meals and make them more enjoyable. Try grocery shopping with a friend, cooking ahead, and freezing portions to have healthy and easy meals on hand, rinse canned vegetables to lower salt content, drain canned fruit to get rid of excess sugars, try new recipes or different herbs and spices, and eat with a friend on occasion. Good nutrition can modify the negative effects of aging by reducing the risk of many chronic diseases, helping you move better, and keeping you mentally sharp. As a result of your physical and mental well-being, you'll be much more able to cope with the stress in your life.

Coping with Middle Age

It's been the brunt of jokes for years, but it can become a serious matter when someone is going through a "midlife crisis." At the age of thirty, middle age still seems like a long ways away, but by the time we reach forty, it finally hits us that we're at the midpoint of our lives. For many of us, that fortieth birthday can be a very traumatic period of life.

One of the tragedies of middle age is the rising suicide rate among adults aged thirty-five to sixty-four. Annual suicide rates for this age group increased 28 percent between 1999 and 2010, with particularly high increases among non-Hispanic whites and American Indians and Alaska natives. The key findings by the CDC were as follows:

- Suicide rates among those thirty-five to sixty-four-years old increased 32 percent for women and 27 percent for men.

- The greatest increases in suicide rates were among people aged fifty to fifty-four years (48 percent) and fifty-five to fifty-nine years (49 percent).

Suicide rates increased 23 percent or more across all four major regions of the United States. Individuals seem to react differently to finding themselves in middle age, and sometimes the differences are related to gender. While a man may experience feelings of inadequacy and depression because he feels as if his life and career are not where he thought they would be at this stage, a woman may actually experience more happiness and fulfillment now that her children no longer need so much attention. Or vice versa. Like everything else, the reaction depends upon the individual. The good news is that even though men and women may begin midlife differently, evidence shows they both end up discovering greater happiness and life satisfaction as they grow older. By the time they reach the age of sixty-five, men and women have usually gone through the worst periods of midlife and begin to enjoy their lives again.

The key to getting through that forty- to sixty-four-year-old period is to stay productive and try to do the things you've always wanted to do. Rather than grumble about getting older and being in a rut, think of middle age as a perfect time to experience different things, expand your horizons by learning something new, and explore exciting opportunities. To approach midlife with a whole new set of attitudes, here are some suggestions:

- **Never stop learning.** One of the main reasons that people go through midlife crises is that they take to heart the adage that you can't teach an old dog new tricks. That's simply not the case. To keep yourself feeling young at heart, learn a musical instrument, take up a new hobby, or go back to school if you feel like you're in a rut or want a new career. The happiest midlifers are the ones who never think they're over-the-hill and instead make plans for what may be their most productive years.

- **Keep active.** One of the biggest obstacles to a happy and vibrant midlife is thinking that it's all behind us and that we have nothing left to offer. The best way to overcome that is to stay active in whatever interests you, whether its politics, social causes, charities, or volunteer work. Keeping active outside work will add new meaning to your life and help get you through those critical middle years.

- **Plan ahead.** If you want to do all of the things you dreamed of doing when you were younger, you need the resources that allow you the freedom to pursue them.

By planning ahead, you'll look forward to your future as a time of new and continued opportunities and great possibilities.

- **Eat right and stay fit.** When both men and women reach middle age, biological changes begin to occur that are made worse by poor nutrition and inactivity. Eating well, maintaining a healthy weight, and exercising regularly will do wonders for both physical and mental health.

- **Stop and smell the roses.** Midlife is the time to reflect on all the big and little things you've accomplished thus far. You still have half a lifetime to accomplish even more. Take advantage of this time by traveling, meeting new friends, and enjoying life.

Most of us set out on a career path—sometimes the wrong career path—without really exploring or developing our hidden talents. And when we go through life doing only what we've been trained to do, we begin to question whether or not there's more to accomplish. Psychologists tell us that there are two kinds of people who tend to avoid midlife crises: those who believe that they have fulfilled many of their life's dreams and goals by the time they reach forty, and those who live in the moment, don't worry so much about the past, and find happiness in today. Most of us don't fit either category, so we need to do a better job of coping with the fact that we've reached middle age. The best way to avoid crisis during those middle years is to develop what psychologists call our shadow side in order to reach our full potential and feel truly satisfied that we've become all we can be.

Coping with Grief

As we age, we naturally experience more losses and, with them, more grief. More of our friends and family get sick or die. We see our parents and ourselves growing older, and the realization of our own mortality comes home to us. Illness and death are very stressful life events for anyone who has to care for a loved one as he or she goes through such a traumatic process. If we don't cope well with crises in general, we'll certainly have trouble dealing with the illness or death of someone close to us; and our depressed immune system will certainly make us more susceptible to disease. It's not uncommon for individuals to become seriously ill shortly after the death of a spouse. To help you cope better with grief, here are four effective techniques:

1. **Don't keep emotions bottled up.** Expressing emotions is part of a healthy grieving process, so don't suppress them just for the sake of appearing strong. Grieving can last for months, but some individuals go through periods of grief for years even after resuming a normal life. Expressing feelings and allowing the normal grieving process to take its course will help you resume a healthy and emotionally satisfying life.

2. **Don't grieve by yourself.** Grief can go on for a long time if we keep others from helping us get through it. It's easy to become withdrawn and lonely when we feel that no one can understand what we're going through. Allowing others to give us some comfort, even if it's with a dinner or a brief visit, can help us cope much better with stress and at least get us back to a normal routine.

3. **Get counseling if grief becomes overwhelming.** For those suffering from "pathologic grief," bereavement becomes a seemingly permanent process that may last a year or more. If you find yourself suffering from severe anxiety or depression, or if your grief is causing more serious emotional problems, seek professional help before your emotional issues trigger chronic illness or disease.

4. **Do things to get your mind off your grief.** After a reasonable period of time, get away and do whatever takes your mind away from the source of grief. Schedule

dinners with family and friends, go to a movie, or become active in social or volunteer groups. Anything that occupies your time and helps you fill the void will speed up your recovery and prevent the emotional pain that becomes debilitating if isn't dealt with at the outset. However, avoid self-medicating with alcohol or other drugs as much as possible.

If your friends or loved ones are grieving, don't sit on the sidelines; offer them help and support in getting through their grief. Remember, while you may not be able to ease their pain, you can still help them cope and make life a little more manageable. Just being there, listening, holding their hand, or talking will give them solace and make recovery less painful. And by actively helping them, you will be helping yourself, as well. Activity is the great antidote to depression.

Aging and Mental Health

It's estimated that 20 percent of people aged fifty-five years or older will experience some type of mental health issue. The most common conditions include anxiety, cognitive impairment, and depression. Mental health issues often contribute to suicide, with older men having the highest suicide rate of any age group. In fact, men aged eighty-five years or older have a suicide rate of forty-five per 100,000, compared to an overall rate of eleven per 100,000 for all ages.

Depression is the most common mental health problem among older adults and is typically associated with distress and suffering, which then leads to impairments in physical, mental, and social functioning. Depression can also decrease immune function and significantly affect the treatment of other chronic diseases. Older adults with depression pay more visits to doctors, use more medications, and have longer hospital stays. Although the rate of depression tends to increase with age, depression is not a normal part of aging. Rather, in

80 percent of cases it is a treatable condition. Unfortunately, depression in older adults is widely under-recognized and often untreated.

The good news is that the majority of older adults do not have mental health issues. Older brains, if used regularly, can actually regenerate nerve cells and stimulate growth of nerve networks. In fact, researchers have found that diseases like Alzheimer's can be slowed down simply by reading, working puzzles, and solving problems, and that certain intellectual functions that rely on the application of learned material remain intact well into our seventies. At the University of Southern California, a twenty-one-year-long study of people twenty-two to eighty-one years old found that intellectual competence was maintained or actually improved as the individuals got older. More surprising was the fact that 10 percent of subjects in their seventies actually performed better than they had ten or even twenty years earlier.

Attempting to explain why older brains could perform so well, researchers at the University of Rochester discovered that the cortex of aged brains had more extensive nerve fibers than did younger brains. Since nerve fibers in the cortex provide information to brain areas responsible for learning and memory, the researchers concluded that, as long as the brain remains healthy, the capacity for analyzing and processing information continues well into old age. As yet, no one knows the age at which nerves in a healthy brain begin to die more quickly than they are replaced, since the oldest brain studied was ninety-two years old and still had an extensive network of nerve fibers.

More recently, in one of the most remarkable studies done, researchers at Princeton University have presented the final piece of evidence. Until now, it was thought that our brain would grow lots of neural connections early in life; but as we aged, our brain cells would gradually die and be lost forever. What the Princeton brain research team discovered for the first time was the neural pathway responsible for reasoning, intelligence, and thinking. And what they saw was that neurons in mature brains have a natural mechanism that regenerates and repopulates neurons so that they can be replaced as quickly as they are lost.[18]

What these studies have shown is that neural connections continue to grow, and that intelligence doesn't have to decline with age, as long as the brain remains healthy. In some cases it actually gets better, confirming that the ability to learn and remember is really a lifelong process. To slow brain aging and keep those neurons regenerating, it's important to remain physically and mentally active. Nothing is worse for the brain than a poor cardiovascular system that doesn't bring enough oxygen to brain cells.

If you need proof that age is simply a number, just look at some of the greatest writers, painters, musicians, scientists, and scholars in history who have done their best work well into their seventies. We should follow their example and never allow age to get in the way of our ambitions, dreams, or goals. Here are some suggestions on how we can improve brain function, creativity, and memory well into old age.

- **Stimulate the brain.** Just like the muscles in your body need to be worked out so they don't atrophy, the brain needs to be worked out as well. Stimulating brain cells by working puzzles, reading, playing a musical instrument, or learning new hobbies triggers growth of neural connections and prevents memory loss. While in his eighties, my father would work algebra problems for an hour each day to keep his brain conditioned. In my opinion, his mind was as sharp when he died at eighty-six as it was when he was younger simply because he exercised it every single day.

- **Exercise at least three times a week.** The brain needs oxygen in order to function and to regenerate. Exercising to the point that you increase heart rate sends a flood of oxygenated blood to the brain, which then repairs damaged cells and builds new ones. Older individuals don't need to work out like Olympic athletes. Moderate exercise like walking thirty minutes a day or doing a few laps in the swimming pool is enough to work mental health wonders.

• **Eat foods that boost brain power.** According to the latest research, certain foods contain chemicals that increase mental capacity and boost memory. These brain-healthy foods increase blood flow to the brain by reducing plaque building cholesterol and decreasing the risk of heart disease and diabetes. The best foods for boosting brain power are apples, blackberries, goji berries, dark chocolate, oatmeal, beans, extra virgin olive oil, salmon, walnuts, and Concord grape juice.

• **Use herbal supplements to boost memory.** Throughout the world, and for centuries, herbs have been used by local populations to keep the brain healthy. When you look at populations that have the healthiest brains in the elderly and the lowest rates of dementia, you find that these individuals consume lots of turmeric, cinnamon, flaxseed, rosemary, ginger, basil, and ginkgo biloba.

• **Get enough brain vitamins.** There are four vitamins known to increase brain power and short term memory: 1. **Folic acid**, found in leafy green vegetables and legumes, repairs damaged brain cells and enhances alertness; 2. **Vitamin B12**, found in poultry, fish, pork, and beef, maintains healthy nerve cells and helps manufacture myelin, the fatty sheath that surrounds nerves and is critical for nerve transmission; 3. **Vitamin C**, found in a variety of fruits and vegetables, is a powerful antioxidant that eliminates free radicals, molecules that can damage brain cells; and 4. **Vitamin E**, found in leafy green vegetables, nuts, and grains, is another powerful antioxidant that eliminates free radicals. Researchers have found that older individuals who took Vitamin E supplements delayed and even prevented Alzheimer's disease altogether.

- **Get at least seven hours of sleep.** Many sleep experts claim that sleep is the number one step older individuals should take to improve memory. According to research, the brain is rejuvenated and the growth of neural connections is sped up during sleep. Even naps are beneficial, so if you're not getting your seven to eight hours of sleep a night, make sure you nap sometime during the day.

- **Be aware of drug interactions.** As you age, it's important to be aware that more use of medicines and normal body changes caused by aging can increase the chance of unwanted or even harmful drug interactions. For example, changes in the digestive system can affect how fast medicines enter the bloodstream. Changes in body weight can influence the amount of medicine you need to take and how long it stays in your body. The circulatory system may slow down and affect how fast drugs get to the liver and kidneys. The liver and kidneys may work more slowly and affect the way a drug breaks down and is removed from the body. All these factors can alter an individual's senses and mental capacity.

- **Get a regular health checkup.** In many cases, memory and mental capacity are directly linked to a physical health problem such as low or high hormone levels, anemia, blood pressure, or blood flow. All of these are easily measured and can be treated. If a mental health issue is related to a physical problem, the solution may be as simple as a prescription medication.

- **De-stress, even if it's only a few minutes a day.** It's amazing just how severely stress can affect one's brain. Physical and emotional stress not only saps our energy levels, it depresses immunity, disrupts the mind-body connection, and sometimes makes us seem as though we're in a fog. To reverse that brain drain, take some time out to go on a trip or simply enjoy the solitude of a quiet walk.

Medication and the Mind-Body Connection

Although food and drug interactions can occur in people of all ages, they pose special problems for the elderly, who are major users of prescription and over-the-counter drugs. More than half the elderly take at least one medication a day; some take five or more. What's more significant is that they're less likely than younger patients to be well-informed about how and when to take these drugs. The side effects can lead to confusion and severe emotional stress because the mind and body may react in a negative and often alarming way.

Certain drugs may also promote dietary deficiencies. Antacids containing aluminum hydroxide, for example, may contribute to phosphate deficiency. Aspirin can cause small amounts of bleeding in the gastrointestinal tract and lead to iron depletion. Laxatives affect vitamin D absorption and calcium balance. And mineral oil can interfere with absorption of vitamins A, D, E, and K and can also interfere with anticoagulants.

Surveys show that older patients are often lacking information about the medicines they're prescribed. Those who take three or more different medications at the same time should be especially cautious. The best way for the elderly to begin taking responsibility for their use of medication is to ask themselves the following questions and discuss these issues with their medical providers.

- Does the medication make me feel worse than the illness itself? If so, have I reported any adverse reactions to my physician immediately?

- Am I taking medications only upon medical advice and under a physician's supervision, not on the advice of relatives or friends?

- Is my personality or physical condition being negatively altered when I add another medication to my usage?

- Can one medication be substituted for another so as to eliminate any adverse side effects?

- Am I taking the minimum dosage that's required?

- Am I taking a few medications well instead of many that cause confusion and improper usage?

- Do I discontinue using a medication when it's no longer required? Is the medication I'm taking really necessary?

- Do I clean out my medicine cabinet regularly and discard any old medicines? Are all medicine bottles labeled in large, clear letters? Do I take medicines only after checking the labels carefully and, at night, only with the light on?

- Do I carry with me information about medications or other special treatment being used, as well as my physician's name and telephone number? Do I have a list of all medications and dosages I'm taking to show my doctor or pharmacist if I ever need to?

The aim of drug (medication) treatment is to cure disease, relieve symptoms, and improve organ function. But because we all respond differently to drugs over the course of our lifespan, we need to be more aware of drug reactions and accept the fact that as we age we become more sensitive than ever to food-drug interactions. By misusing or overusing medications, we may actually be interfering with how the mind-body connection works. And the last thing we need as we go through the aging process is for the treatment to be worse than the illnesses we get.

Medications That Deplete Nutrients

As you age, chances are that you'll be taking one or more medications, some of which can rob you of vital nutrients that affect both mind and body. The most common ones are beta blockers and vasodilators for heart problems, statins for cholesterol, diuretics for high blood pressure and congestive heart failure, and hormone therapy for menopause and other hormonal imbalances. Because the vast majority of seniors take at least one drug on a regular basis, one of the best ways to counteract this hidden side effect and avoid nutrient imbalance is to eat certain foods and take specific supplements. Here are four ways to do that.

1. **Beta blockers and vasodilators.** These drugs tend to deplete the body of coenzyme Q10, which is responsible for supplying 95 percent of the energy needed for metabolic processes, and vitamin B6, which plays a key role in a multitude of biochemical reactions. Foods with the highest levels of coQ10 are fish, beef liver, and eggs. B6 is found in whole grains, poultry, fish, fruits, vegetables, and legumes. It may also be a good idea to add a coQ10 supplement, especially if you're taking statin drugs.

2. **Statins.** Statins also have been known to deplete coenzyme Q10. Although these drugs do a great job of lowering cholesterol, patients often complain about muscle pain and fatigue. If you're on a statin, ask your doctor about supplementing with 100 mg of coQ10 daily. In addition, you need to be adding fish, lean meat, and poultry to your diet. (Many people taking beta blockers are also taking statins; if you are one of them, it may be especially important to ask your doctor about supplementing coQ10.)

3. **Diuretics.** Used to treat people with high blood pressure and congestive heart failure, diuretics, which cause

you to urinate frequently, tend to deplete the body of magnesium, potassium, and zinc. All three of these vital minerals are important in a variety of life functions such as heart rate, nerve conduction, muscle contraction, and immune function. To counteract these losses, eat dark leafy greens, nuts, whole grains, and beans for magnesium; apricots, raisins, nuts, and bananas for potassium; and roasted pumpkin seeds, peanuts, dark chocolate, and lean roast beef for zinc. As a supplement, 8 mg of zinc for women and 11 mg for men is a good dose. For magnesium, 400 mg is standard.

4. **Hormone Therapy.** Many women, and quite a few men, are on some kind of hormone or hormone replacement therapy. These can deplete the body of vitamin C, vitamin B6, zinc, and magnesium, as well as folate. To counter these effects, eat lots of fruits, green leafy vegetables, and whole grains. It's also a good idea to include a supplement with vitamins, folic acid, magnesium, and zinc as well.

Strength Training for Seniors

While it's true that muscle begins to decrease as one gets older, in many cases it's because of inactivity. There's no reason that an individual can't maintain good strength well into old age, especially if he or she works out at least three times a week using weight-bearing exercises. As an example, I compete in the senior Olympics and can lift twice as much weight today than I ever could twenty or thirty years ago because I began a routine strength training program. Muscles respond to stimuli regardless of their age.

Before you start throwing heavy barbells around, it's always a smart idea to get a checkup and get clearance from your doctor. After you do, begin slowly so that your muscles adjust to their new activity. To get the most from your strength training and new muscle growth, here are some tips for older individuals.

- Lift heavy enough that you can't get more than eight to twelve reps. Anything more than that and you're really just training for endurance.

- Focus on multiple joint exercises like bench press, squats, deadlifts, and overhead press rather than isolation exercises like bicep curls. Multiple joint exercises work several muscle groups together and give you more bang for the buck. Chin-ups and pushups are also great multi-joint exercises.

- Take a day off between workouts to allow your muscles to recover and grow. Remember, muscle growth occurs when you rest, not when you exercise.

- Consume protein with every meal. Protein is what builds muscle, so if you can't get enough protein with meals, add a protein shake every day.

- Get a good night's sleep. Your muscles grow when you sleep, so it's important to get in at least seven hours.

Special Health Tips for Aging Successfully

As we've seen, physiological events during aging alter mind-body networks and increase the likelihood of stress-related illness and disease. Consequently, elderly individuals have to recognize and deal with stressors to which they, as a group, are especially susceptible. Successful aging depends not only on good health habits but also on coping strategies that deal with loneliness, physical disability, rejection, and feelings of worthlessness. These emotional stresses are so powerful that older people may find it impossible to cope in a society that sees them as a burden.

Personal interactions are an important factor in maintaining physical health and independence because social isolation has been linked to accelerated aging. Elderly who don't participate in social organizations, for example, have much higher rates of disease, whereas elderly who belong to religious or close ethnic groups, or whose families live close by, are much less likely to succumb to stress-related disease. One study found that people lacking social interactions had three times the mortality rate over a ten-year period than people having close social ties.

Social support networks offer an outlet for sharing and interacting, and they enrich our lives by making us feel useful and needed and by giving us a sense of dignity. Aging, after all, doesn't mean an end to our challenges but the beginning of a new phase of life in which we can fulfill those challenges in different but equally satisfying ways. The biggest hurdles many seniors face is the gradual breakdown in immunity, increased frequency of illness, and negative attitudes that life is all but over and/or that it didn't turn out the way we thought it would or should. The following are effective mind-body strategies that can help older people overcome those attitudes, deal with the stress in their lives and, consequently, slow down the aging process.

- **Expand your horizons.** Human needs go beyond survival and subsistence. Look to enjoy old and establish new interests, develop new activities, learn, and make contributions to others. Participating in classes, clubs, and enrichment programs is a great way to increase self-esteem and achieve something worthwhile.

- **Stay active.** A key factor in maintaining a positive connection between mind and body is the satisfying and constructive use of leisure time. When that time also involves sports activities, it becomes an important contributing factor in health, vitality, and longevity. Endurance exercises like walking, for instance, improve the body's sensitivity to insulin. In fact, walking forty minutes a day can cut the risk of type 2 diabetes by 40 percent, and stretching that out to an hour can cut the risk in half. Exercise also helps us shed pounds, boosts energy reserves, and triggers release of endorphins, which help us cope with physical and emotional stress.

- **Keep up with your health care.** Older people tend to view minor health problems as normal to aging and, thus, often fail to get adequate medical treatment. Minor health problems then lead to major health disorders, which create intense physical and emotional stress situations. It's also important to recognize mental health problems just as you would any other health disorder. Self-deprecation, loss of appetite, and insomnia (especially awakening in the early morning hours) may be symptoms of clinical depression, not aging. Never assume that any kind of physical or mental illness is a normal by-product of aging.

- **Know your medications.** As we get older and take more medications, our bodies will not respond in the same way as when we were younger. Don't hesitate to ask your doctor and pharmacist about side effects, interactions with foods and other drugs, and the effectiveness of generic alternatives. The more you know, the better off you'll be.

- **Eat well.** Research programs around the country have shown that consuming the required nutrients, reducing high-fat foods and cutting down on calories has an anti-aging effect on the body. Eating right doesn't necessarily mean that you'll live longer if you're genetically predisposed to some sort of health problem; it does mean that you'll experience fewer stress reactions, have a stronger and healthier immune system, and live a lot better as you grow older. To ensure that you're covering all the nutritional bases, eat beans for fiber, fish for omega-3, nuts for healthy fats, berries for antioxidants, dark leafy greens for vitamins and minerals, and whole grains for blood sugar control.

- **Give up bad habits.** Smoking and excess alcohol consumption is bad enough at any age, but for older people they can be especially deadly. Nicotine and other tobacco ingredients speed up metabolism of certain drugs. Alcohol causes changes in the liver, which can also speed up metabolism of drugs such as anticonvulsants, anticoagulants, and diabetes medications. These drugs become less effective because they either don't stay in the body long enough or are altered in some way. For example, if alcohol abuse damages the liver a drug can remain in the body too long and cause damage. Smoking and alcohol abuse, then, can bring on physical health problems not only by their own actions but also by their interactions with medications. Adverse drug reactions then lead to negative stress responses that encourage even more smoking and drinking.

- **Get a pet.** It's well known that talking to and stroking animals can decrease blood pressure, and that owning a pet can improve the chances of surviving a heart attack. Animals, especially pets such as dogs and cats, can greatly enhance an older person's physical and emotional health by combating depression and loneliness and reducing the effects of stress. Pets are good medicine because they satisfy needs such as caring and a desire to be loved and needed. According to experts, as older people withdraw from human affairs, their nonhuman environment becomes even more important. Animals fulfill the human craving for emotional relationships and promote interactions and involvement.

- **Do everything in moderation.** People who live to an old age and stay healthy tend to limit their stress responses, eat right, limit their calorie intake (1800 calories a day compared with the average Western diet of 3300 calories a day), and lead a simple and healthy lifestyle that includes limiting their tobacco and alcohol use. They consume foods high in fiber (plenty of fruits and vegetables) and low in saturated fats. They also continue to work or keep active; tend not to worry about their age; and maintain friendships and involvement in social support networks.

- **Learn relaxation exercises.** A study of elderly people living in retirement homes showed that those who practiced relaxation exercises had significant increases in natural killer cell activity and significant decreases in antibodies to herpes simplex virus—both indicators of enhanced immune activity.[19] This is especially important since immune function and the ability to fend off stress-related illnesses decrease with age.

- **Seek out social support.** As we age, it becomes more and more important to develop a network of friends and family. Becoming isolated after we retire or after our spouse dies is easy. Before we know it, we lose contacts, get comfortable staying home, and find it harder and harder to become stimulated. To prevent loneliness and depression from setting in, make it a habit to get out every day. Take up a hobby that includes contact with other people. And make it a point to see family regularly and often—in-person, if at all possible, or through video chatting via the Internet.

Research has now shown that aging is indeed accelerated by physical and emotional stress, unhealthy lifestyles, and poor nutrition, all of which combine to disrupt the mind-body connection, depress immunity, and cause a breakdown in homeostasis. As we age, it becomes all the more important to prevent the symptoms of stress reactions and not treat them simply as symptoms of aging. By adopting a healthy lifestyle, keeping active, and practicing relaxation exercises, we can slow aging and live out our lives in the healthiest way possible.

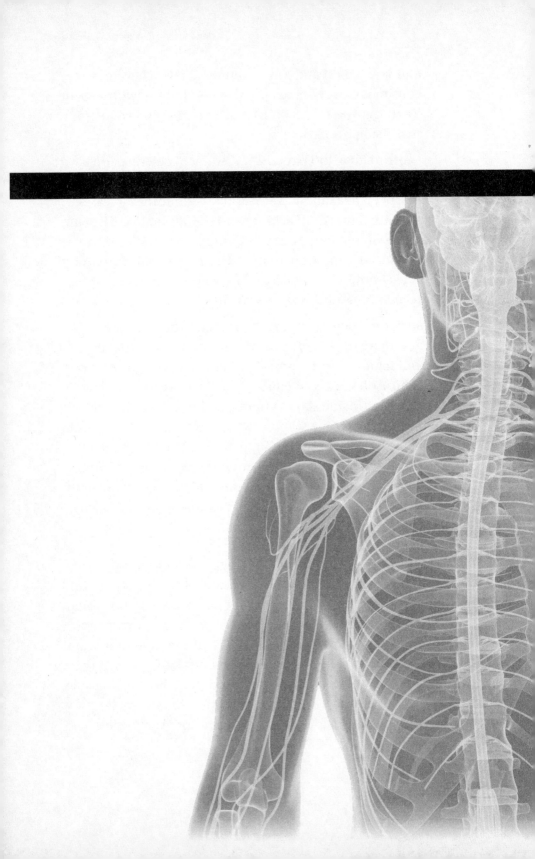

CHAPTER SEVEN

Meditation

An Ancient Practice Perfect for Modern Life

For centuries, meditation has been the method of choice for inducing relaxation and achieving peace of mind. In fact, Eastern medicine has known all along what the West is only now beginning to understand: that the mind and body cannot be separated, and that meditation is a powerful tool in helping the mind trigger the hormonal responses needed to achieve a healthier body. Since our mind is the connective force between the various systems of the body, meditation is a way to bring all those systems into harmony and equilibrium.

The term meditation refers to a mind-body practice that increases calmness and physical relaxation, improves psychological balance, and enhances overall wellness. Though various cultures and religious groups have practiced it in one form or another, meditation in itself is neither a religion nor a philosophy. Rather, it's a tool that uses the conditioning power of the brain to evoke relaxation, tranquility, and inner peace. The end result is both a decrease in negative stress reactions and a triggering of what's been called the "relaxation response." It's through a decrease in the body's stress reactions that we boost our immune system and keep our body healthy and disease-free.

In Western cultures, meditation often incorporates vocals such as Gregorian chants, repetitive words, as used by Catholics in reciting the Hail Mary on rosary beads, incantations from the Hebrew Kabbalah, and spiritual chants used by Native Americans. All of these techniques are aimed at achieving a deep state of awareness and, at the same time, using the power of the mind to succumb to relaxation.

We've made a complete circle in the way we think about the effects of meditation on health. In the distant past, the concept of a mind-body connection was accepted as a foregone conclusion. People meditated because they knew that healing the body required healing the soul as well. During the last century, though, scientists and physicians, as well as companies marketing an explosion of newly developed drugs and medicines, had us convinced that the body is simply a machine that needs repair when it breaks or wears down. The power of the mind to trigger healing was largely discounted until newly educated scientists actually began testing practitioners of meditation and found that mind over matter is not just an expression but a medical fact of life.

How Meditation Works

There are several different forms of meditation, most of which originated in ancient religious and spiritual traditions. The two most common types are mindfulness meditation, which is an essential component of Zen Buddhism, and transcendental meditation (TM), derived from Hindu traditions. In both types, the person achieves a state of deeply relaxed awareness. The main difference is that in mindfulness meditation, the individual's attention is on breathing and focusing on what is being experienced while in transcendental meditation, the focus is on a mantra that prevents distracting thoughts from entering the mind.

Meditation connects the mind and body by inducing physical changes that affect the involuntary or autonomic nervous system (ANS). This system regulates many organs and muscles, and it affects functions such as heartbeat, breathing, digestion, and sweating. The sympathetic division of the ANS triggers the "fight-or-flight response," which increases heart rate, breathing, and blood flow whenever we're stressed. The parasympathetic division does the opposite; it decreases heart rate and breathing, and causes us to slow down (Figure 7.1). Practicing meditation reduces activity in the sympathetic division and increases activity in the parasympathetic division.

Figure 7.1: The Functions of the Autonomic Nervous System

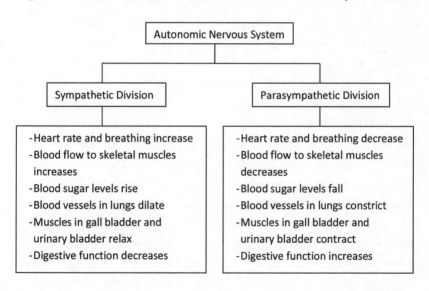

One of the main reasons that meditation has been around for at least 5,000 years is that, at its core, it's very simple. There's no need for tools or sophisticated gadgets. And an individual can meditate alone and just about anywhere he or she chooses.

In essence, meditation works because it relies on the untapped power of the brain to guide the body processes responsible for mental, emotional, and physical cleansing.

The benefits of meditation start almost immediately. Stress and anxiety are reduced, heart rate is decreased, blood pressure is lowered, immunity is enhanced, and energy levels are boosted. When blood is drawn from individuals who are meditating, it typically has a significantly lower ESR (erythrocyte sedimentation rate), a test that indicates the likelihood of disease, illness, or infection. The guidelines for proper meditation described below enhance these effects and make the experience much more effective and enjoyable. Adhering to these guidelines from the outset ensures that meditation works the way it's supposed to.

Meditation and the Mind-Body Connection

The beauty of meditation lies in its simplicity. Allow the mind to free itself of negative thoughts and conditioning and the body will respond by automatically relaxing, healing, and rejuvenating itself in the process. It goes beyond that, though. The act of meditation has a profound effect on the mind-body connection, changing brainwave patterns and specifically enhancing alpha brain waves, which promote health and self-healing. Furthermore, meditation lowers blood levels of cortisol, the main hormone involved in negative stress reactions and susceptibility to disease.

One of the first to use meditation as a means of balancing the body's physiological processes was Herbert Benson, MD, Director of the Mind-Body Institute at Harvard Medical School, who, in 1969, found that meditation countered the effects of the sympathetic nervous system involved in the fight-or-flight response. He observed decreased muscle tension, blood pressure, body temperature, and basal metabolic rate. In general, the patients who meditated had healthier immune systems and recovered more quickly when they *did* get sick.

Since Dr. Benson's pioneering efforts, others have shown similar results. Researchers at the Biofeedback and Psychophysiology Clinic at the Menninger Foundation have demonstrated that cancer and AIDS patients had stronger immune systems when they used meditative techniques either alone or in conjunction with biofeedback. Dean Ornish, MD, the famous heart surgeon, found that heart disease could be reversed with a comprehensive program that includes meditation. Because of these remarkable findings, over six thousand physicians now practice meditation and recommend it to their patients.

Based on two decades of clinical studies, we know that meditation affects virtually every part of the body. The mind-body network is mobilized into action and conditioned to bring the two into balance. Besides stress relief, meditation has been shown to reduce pain, slow tumor growth, reverse heart disease, lower blood pressure, treat insomnia, lower cholesterol, increase fertility, moderate asthma, reduce PMS and migraines, and treat fibromyalgia. The psychological benefits include decreased anxiety and depression, and enhanced mood, concentration, and learning.

In a new study, researchers at Massachusetts General Hospital, the University of Arizona, Boston University, and Emory University found that the effects of meditation last well beyond the time that you're actually practicing it. What researchers saw was that activity in the brain's amygdala, the part of the brain responsible for emotional reactions, decreased in response to stress and negative life events after taking an eight-week course in meditation.[20] This was the first time that meditation was shown to affect emotional response even when a person is not in a meditative state. The results of the study are profound in that we now know for certain that meditation is not just an immediate reaction that lasts for the duration of the exercise but is a long-term response that enables one to cope with stress and negative emotions throughout the day.

The body doesn't really care how the mind does it, as long as the results are effective and long-lasting. Whether meditation is through prayer, mindfulness meditation, transcendental meditation, Zen meditation, Buddhist meditation, or Taoist meditation doesn't matter. All these practices have three things in common: (1) quieting of the busy mind; (2) focusing concentration on a sound, word, image, or breath; and (3) directing the body to fall into a deeply relaxed state. According to Joan Borysenko, PhD, author of *Minding the Body, Mending the Mind*, "Meditation can put one in touch with the inner physician, allowing the body's own inner wisdom to be heard."[21]

Four Rules of Meditation

Stress researchers who have studied the effects of meditation on body functions, mental health, and the relaxation response have found that four basic elements are necessary for achieving a state of deep relaxation. They are:

1. **A quiet space.** Meditation, like other stress management techniques, is most effective when you're free of distractions. And since concentration is the most basic component of meditation, make sure that wherever you choose to meditate is quiet and peaceful for the duration of the exercise. A quiet room or a peaceful backyard can be the perfect place to meditate as long as you're not disturbed.

2. **A comfortable position.** Because any muscle tension can break your concentration, comfort is important. You may assume any position, but the most effective is a sitting position in a chair or on a firm pillow or rug, with your head, neck, and back straight. Lying down is not as effective because many people have a tendency to become too drowsy and fall asleep.

   When assuming the sitting position, don't sit in a way that will cause cramps. The spine should be upright, but not so rigid that you're straining. If you can't sit comfortably with your legs crossed, place your feet flat on the floor and your hands loose and relaxed on your lap. Some people prefer to keep their palms separated and facing up; others like to have one palm resting on the other with the thumbs touching.

3. **A passive state.** Meditation is all about freeing your mind, not guiding your thoughts. Nothing is more distracting during meditation than to have intrusive thoughts. When distractions pop up, disregard them without being too concerned about whether they're affecting your exercise. The worst thing to do at that point is worry about how you're performing. Remain calm and passive and allow distracting thoughts to simply float away. The most effective way to do that is through a mental device or mantra.

4. **A mantra.** To reach a passive state and keep distracting thoughts from interfering with your meditation, focus on a sound, a word, or a phrase, repeated over and over during the exercise. Because total concentration is so difficult to attain, using a mantra allows you to break distracting thoughts and reach a deeper level of internal awareness. Don't choose a mental device that will cause you to think about it rather than on the meditation itself. Rather, choose one that will create a feeling of peace and tranquility that makes you forget about the mechanics of the technique. Whatever mantra you choose—religious expression, sound, a single word— make sure that it's one that frees you from outside forces. Only you can decide, either through practice or by trial and error, what's best and most effective for you.

Naturally, as with any stress management technique, there are some other general guidelines to follow. These are:

- Begin slowly, perhaps five minutes a day before working your way up to fifteen to twenty minutes. There's nothing worse than trying something new and pushing yourself so hard that you quit before you see results.

- When breathing, close your mouth, place your tongue along the roof of the mouth, and breathe smoothly through your nose. Don't force your breathing; just become aware of your breaths as they enter and leave your body. Don't take short or rapid breaths because this will lead to tension. Many meditative exercises include counting your breaths. When you count, always do so as you exhale, softly and quietly.

- If possible, choose a specific time and place to do your meditation. Morning is great because it starts your day; evening is also good because it helps you wind down. In any case, try to meditate regularly, even if you don't feel like it. Five minutes is better than none.

The Importance of Breathing

One of the most important aspects of meditation is proper breathing, because without it meditation becomes nothing more than a fifteen-minute downtime session. In order to maximize the effect of meditation, you must learn to breathe in a way that enhances the link between the respiratory and nervous systems. Scientists have discovered years ago that the manner in which we breathe has a direct effect on the mind-body connection and, consequently, on the various biochemical reactions that influence both physical and mental health. It's the thread that ties together the mind and the body and brings us back into relaxed equilibrium. For this reason, an integral part of any meditative exercise is steady and controlled breathing, which allows our brain to take in more oxygen and actually speeds up the healing process.

Just think about how much breathing is involved with everything we do. From the time we're born to the day we take our last breath, we gasp, yawn, scream, hold our breath, vent our feelings, and sigh with emotion. We whisper to each other, yell at each other, and breathe out to form billions of words in a lifetime. With each breath we take, oxygen nourishes our brain, stimulates cell regeneration, and brings balance between the central nervous and respiratory systems. No other human act we do sustains our life and keeps us as healthy as breathing.

For mediation to work, we need to practice breathing, because it's the act of breathing that helps us achieve a deeply relaxed state. In essence, proper breathing controls the rhythm and flow of meditative exercises, helps keep our mind focused, and maintains our energy levels. The following are the most common types of breathing exercises I teach in my stress management seminars.

Diaphragm Breathing

Close your eyes, place your right hand right above your waist, your left hand on your chest, and begin to breathe slowly, deeply, and rhythmically. Now feel your right hand moving in and out with each breath while your left hand remains steady. This type of breathing keeps the chest muscles from getting too involved and disrupting your meditation; and it will help you relax much faster.

The most important thing to remember is to breathe smoothly and evenly. Concentrate on the tempo—neither too fast nor too slow. The more evenly you breathe, the more your mind and body will respond and the faster you'll begin to relax. Within a week or so, you'll find that diaphragm breathing is not only less work but it feels more natural.

Uneven Breathing

This type of breathing takes a little getting used to because it's not the normal inhalation and exhalation you're used to. Instead of breathing in and out with the same length breaths, you exhale two to three times longer than you inhale. As practice, begin breathing normally and evenly for a minute, and then change the pattern. Inhale for three seconds and exhale for six seconds. Don't focus so much on the time difference as on the breathing itself. Make it smooth and effortless, without pausing between breaths and without worrying about running out of air when you exhale.

Deep Breathing

Breathing deeply is a common technique used to relieve tension. Practiced often enough, it increases your ability to link mind and body, and it leads to a fuller and deeper relaxed state. With this breathing technique, you breathe in slowly for five or six seconds and then hold it for a full ten seconds. Don't think about holding your breathe; just count to yourself and exhale slowly on ten. Take a few regular breaths and then breathe deeply again. Remember to breathe smoothly and evenly without focusing too much on the fact that you're holding your breath.

Mantra Meditation Techniques

There are countless mantra exercises, but they all have one thing in common—they use a device like a word or a sound to trigger the relaxation response. The following are four examples of meditative techniques I suggest in stress seminars. Try them all and then decide, based on your personality type, preferences, and lifestyle, which is best for you. If you're a religious person, you might well choose meditation #2. Whichever technique you choose, always follow the rules of meditation so that you can trigger relaxation with the least amount of effort and distraction.

Mantra Meditation #1

For some people, the simplest type of meditation is the most effective because it requires very little to make it work. In this exercise, sit in a comfortable position, close your eyes, and begin to breathe smoothly and slowly. As you exhale, say the word "relax" to yourself. Let the word flow evenly, and try to feel your muscles becoming more relaxed each time you exhale. Continue the exercise for ten minutes, and when you finish just sit quietly with your eyes open for two or three minutes.

Mantra Meditation #2

This meditative technique uses a repetitive prayer as a mantra. In the fourteenth century, it was known as "The Prayer of the Heart." Begin by sitting in a comfortable position with your eyes closed and your breathing slow, smooth, and even. As you exhale, say the words, "Lord, help me relax," or "God, grant me peace." Continue this for ten minutes, repeating the phrase each time you exhale. You can use any religious phrase you like, depending on your religious preferences. The words you choose really don't matter. The important thing is to use the words or the phrase as a way to focus your mind away from your usual day-to-day concerns and onto your body while feeling yourself relaxing.

Mantra Meditation #3

This classic conditioning technique links breathing and relaxation through a rhythmic sound. For example, adjust a metronome to a setting that mirrors your slow and even breathing pattern. Take a breath each time the metronome makes a beat, and then exhale with the next metronome beat. Every time the metronome beats, say the word "relax" and feel the tension melting away and your muscles relaxing more and more with each exhalation. After doing this exercise for several weeks, your brain will automatically associate the metronome's beats with relaxation. It's the classic Pavlovian response. Your brain will become conditioned to recognize a specific sound as a physiological cue and respond to that sound by subconsciously and instantly triggering the relaxation response.

Mantra Meditation #4

Also known as autosuggestion, this meditation is much like self-induced hypnosis. In this exercise, sit in a comfortable chair, look straight ahead, and breathe deeply and evenly. Beginning with the number ten, count backward softly, one number each time you exhale. As you hear the numbers, feel your body getting more and more relaxed. When you reach the number five, feel your eyelids become heavier and start to close. By the time you get to number one, you should be completely relaxed. Stay in that position and continue to breathe slowly and evenly for ten minutes. When you're done, take a deep breath and open your eyes.

This meditation is very effective in conditioning the brain to associate numbers, which act as cues, with increased relaxation. For example, after a few weeks of practice, for the purpose of meditation your brain may link the number six with your eyes beginning to close, number four may trigger the shoulders and chest to relax, and so forth. The objective is to evoke the relaxation response through mind-body conditioning. Within a matter of weeks, during meditation your body will automatically associate a specific number with a specific body response.

Mindfulness Meditation Techniques

The premise of mindfulness meditation, which is being used by more and more clinicians, is that focusing our attention on a single object and, thus, keeping us anchored in the present moment, will free our mind of negative thoughts about the past and the future. It's all about the here and now. The result, according to leading experts, is that we achieve a mind that is calm and at peace.

At the same time, we're strengthening our mind-body connection by teaching ourselves that harmony and well-being are the normal ways in which the mind is supposed to operate. Unlike mantra meditation, which makes use of a device that clears the mind of thoughts, mindfulness meditation welcomes thoughts. Rather than excluding them, we sit quietly, we observe them, and we embrace them.

Mindfulness Exercise #1

This technique makes use of an everyday object that's in the room. You can take a book, a pen, a cup, or a piece of fruit, for example, and notice everything about it right then at that moment. In this case, pick up an apple and hold it in your fingers. Now look at it, all the while feeling the texture of the skin against your fingers, observing its shades of color and its shape. Does it have bumps? Is it warm? Is it rough or smooth? Is it hard or does it have some softness to it? What does it smell like? What does it taste and feel like when you put a piece in your mouth and swirl it around on your tongue and begin to take bites?

Think about what you experienced as you ate and swallowed the apple. The purpose of this exercise is to train your brain to focus, to become aware of the here and now, and to notice the smallest details that you normally would not notice. With enough practice, you'll automatically become more mindful about different tasks you do throughout the day, which helps keep you in the present so you don't dwell on the past or the future.

Mindfulness Exercise #2

This exercise is similar to the previous one except that you'll focus your attention on an object without actually touching it. The purpose here is to learn how to concentrate. Start out by choosing an object such as a figurine on your coffee table and then taking a few slow breaths to relax. Loosen your arms and place your hands softly in your lap. Once you feel yourself relaxed, begin to look at the figurine as you did with the apple.

Notice the shape and color of the figurine, the curves, the height, the way in which it sits on the table. If your concentration begins to drift, and you start to think about other things, bring your focus back to the statue and try to see the smallest details. The whole point here is observing with awareness. At first, you might only be able to do this for two or three minutes. In time, you'll get much better are focusing for longer periods of time.

Mindfulness Exercise #3

This exercise is a progression from the previous one in that you're focusing on a thought, a feeling, or a sensation you have at the moment rather than on a physical object that you look at. Choose a quiet area in your home, make sure you're wearing loose clothing, and sit in a comfortable chair with your hands folded loosely in your lap. Begin by breathing slowly and rhythmically until you feel relaxed and able to focus on the present moment. Then, whatever your thought or feeling is at that moment, become aware of it without reacting to it in either a positive or a negative way. Keep breathing slowly, using your breaths to help you maintain focus. The point here is to detach yourself from any judgments or analysis and simply notice the thought or feeling in a neutral and objective way. Continue this exercise for ten minutes, take a few deep breaths, and stretch.

You can see how virtually any object, any thought, or any activity, including daily, mundane chores can be used for mindfulness exercises. With a little practice, you can take this to the extreme. As you're cleaning the house, you can focus on the specific chore you're doing at the moment. When you're waiting in line at a grocery store, you can breathe deeply and focus on an item in your shopping cart. When you're eating, you can notice the smell, taste, and texture of the food. And when you're brushing your teeth, you can feel the stiffness of the brush and the smell of the toothpaste. Mindfulness like this is not easy at first. But in a few short weeks, you'll find that your concentration is stronger and you'll be able to focus more easily on whatever you choose.

Labyrinth Walking

A labyrinth is an ancient circular symbol that has been used for centuries as a tool for meditation, prayer, and healing. For many people, it represents a journey toward spiritual growth.

Labyrinths are constructed in different sizes and shapes, and are often associated with churches or spirituality centers.

Although labyrinths are usually constructed of circular paths and are walked, you can simply draw a small one on paper and follow the channels slowly with your index finger. Moving your way along the path from beginning to end several times can be a relaxing experience when done as an occasional exercise. You can build a labyrinth out of rocks in your backyard or visit one at a nearby church, monastery, or other spiritual center.

Getting the Most Benefit from Meditation

Just like your muscles respond to regular training and habit formation, the mind-body connection will respond to meditation and become a powerful force in self-healing once you incorporate it into your daily life. Spending two hours every Saturday meditating will not do it, just like exercising one day a week will not give you anywhere near the results you're after. You have to make it a priority and set aside fifteen minutes a day for meditation. That's all it takes. Fifteen minutes each day will quickly train your mind and your autonomic nervous system to respond in a way that will instantly relieve stress and begin the healing process. Nothing is as effective as establishing a routine.

Another advantage to establishing a routine and meditating every day is that your mind and your body will continue to reap the benefits throughout the day, especially if you start out in the morning. Think about what happens when you exercise. The effects last well into the day and you feel energized and vigorous. If you exercised only on Saturday, you might feel great that day or the next, but by Monday you would get sluggish and fatigued. The same happens with meditation. The more you practice it, the better you get at it, and the greater the benefits are for the mind-body connection.

Meditation is a powerful mind-body exercise and an effective stress management tool because it not only trains us to relax but also helps us focus away from stressful thoughts and feelings. As long as we don't overdo it, meditative exercises are safe and pleasurable; they bring balance to our body and peace to our mind. To paraphrase Dr. Ornish, using meditation may help you surf the uncalm ocean waves.

That's what meditation is all about—learning to ride the waves, so to speak; to relax by evoking the relaxation response through a technique or exercise that conditions the brain and triggers positive homeostatic mechanisms. Meditation has been around for centuries, bringing inner peace and tranquility to people of all religions and philosophies. It does this by helping the mind connect with the body in a way that triggers positive immune responses. We, too, can experience peace, tranquility, and self-healing by using the power of our brain to eliminate the stress in our lives.

CHAPTER EIGHT

Guided Imagery and Self-Healing

Picture This

Guided imagery is nothing new. In fact, throughout history people have been using the power of images to boost the body's ability to heal and rejuvenate itself. Thousands of years ago, shamans were among the first to practice visualization as a way to ward off spirits and cleanse the body. As part of their culture, ancient Greeks such as Aristotle and Hippocrates used guided imagery to heal the body because the imagination was thought of as another organ. Early Christians saw the connection between the mind and the body's ability to heal itself, and, so, they practiced a form of mysticism in which certain prayers or the image of Christ played a role in purification and self-healing.

By the twentieth century, guided imagery had become an accepted technique in medicine to promote healing. The basic premise is to connect the mind and body through the process of thinking in pictures. Guided imagery is now used when treating patients suffering with a variety of disorders.

It is a common and effective form of alternative medicine that is becoming an integral part of treatment and that works even better when combined with traditional medicine. That's because the brain can process images in a way that triggers physical responses throughout our organ systems. When you think about how many images go through your mind each day, it's astounding. Virtually every second of your life, you're flooded with thoughts and images from your past, from what you're doing right now, and from what you'll be doing in the future. Many of those images might be negative, in which case the cumulative effect on the body will result in weakened immunity and, eventually, illness and disease. So learning how to control those images and make them work for you can be as powerful a tool as taking medication or undergoing surgery.

How Guided Imagery Works

Watch a top athlete and see how he or she uses visualization to improve performance. In the last Olympics, I observed how hurdlers would look down the track and imagine how they were going to run, how many strides they would need before they got to each hurdle, and how they would leap across the hurdles at precisely the right moment. They would do this over and over again until it was time to get on the starting blocks. Golfers do the same thing. Before each swing, they imagine the flight of the ball and where it will land on the fairway or the green. I find that this really helps me whenever I'm on the golf course.

If you think about what you do each day, you realize that much of your life is spent planning. You plan what you're going to wear, what you'll have for breakfast, what your tasks will be for the next few hours, where lunch will be, what you're going to do for dinner, etc. All this planning goes on inside your head, where you're imagining these things and working out the details. In other words, your life is basically spent visualizing.

Like the athletes I mentioned, we're all natural visualizers in that most everything we do, we see in our minds first. So it's not much of a stretch to say that guided imagery is easy and effective because it's a part of who we are.

Where we tend to get into trouble is that whenever we encounter a problem or experience a stressful situation, many of us tend to over-analyze. Rather than use the power of our imagination, we depend on analytical thinking. And instead of relieving our stress or managing our illness, we make things worse because we allow our negative emotions to take charge and short circuit the mind-body connection. As a result, we can't take advantage of the powerful reactions that stimulate healing. Doing this repeatedly only strengthens the negative conditioning process and weakens our ability to bring our body back into equilibrium

Guided imagery or visualization uses mental pictures, thoughts, symbols, and sensations as a means of achieving a deeply relaxed state. Vivid images associated with rest, tranquility, and serenity are used as positive feedback messages for the rest of the body. These images act as cues that stimulate the nervous system and cause tense muscles to respond subconsciously. Once practiced, guided imagery is one of the simplest and most enjoyable of all relaxation techniques. And like other relaxation exercises, it acts as a tool for triggering the relaxation response—in this case by conditioning the brain to associate mental images with relaxation.

Because of the strong connection between mind and body, guided imagery has been used as a method for inducing self-healing. Its ability to stimulate and strengthen the immune system has been effective in treating various types of cancers and other diseases linked to a breakdown in immune response. In combination with radiation or chemotherapy, guided imagery has resulted in reduction of tumors and higher survival rates than with the use of standard treatments alone. As a result, physicians are recognizing that self-healing is more likely when the power of the brain is used to boost the immune system during those times when it's needed most.

An unexpectedly surprising effect of guided imagery has been with cancer patients. In combination with standard treatment, guided imagery has resulted in reduction of tumors and higher survival rates than with the use of chemotherapy or radiation alone. When a group of elderly people used guided imagery three times a week for a month, their NK cells (cells that seek out and destroy cancer) and T cell counts increased significantly.[22] Similar results with other patients have convinced doctors that curing diseases is more likely when the immune system gets help from a variety of sources.

A probable explanation for the success of guided imagery may be that it reduces cortisol, which triggers a cascade of reactions that leads to depressed immune function and, consequently, to a host of diseases. One study, reported in *Health Psychology*, found that after thirteen weeks of guided imagery, subjects dramatically elevated their mood and significantly reduced their blood cortisol levels, which naturally made them less prone to disease.[23]

Learning to Visualize

Before you can walk or run, you first learn how to take steps. Before you practice guided imagery, you need to learn how to use your imagination to visualize. This takes creativity and the ability to actually see details in your mind. Later in the chapter, when we get to guided imagery for self-healing, this will become even more important.

You might think you're not very good at visualizing, but if you consider that dreams are nothing more than visualizations, you realize that everyone has the ability to imagine just about anything. The difference is that when you dream, your mind is free and uninhibited. So allow your mind to drift and to allow it to use its power to create vivid images. The following are some exercises you can do to strengthen your visualization skills, beginning with the simplest type. Before you begin, make sure that you're comfortable, that you're wearing loose-fitting clothing, and that you're relaxed.

Step One: Visualizing a simple object

Close your eyes, take a few deep breaths, and imagine a single object like a flower. Don't just try to imagine any flower. Make sure you choose one that's very familiar to you so that you can actually see it and describe it. Imagine the flower floating in the air in front of you. Observe the color—is it white, red, or yellow? Are the petals soft or rough? Try to feel the texture of the petals and then move down to the sepal and the stem. Does the flower have a round shape? Is it long or is it asymmetrical? Now smell the flower. Does it smell sweet or pungent? Continue to observe the details for a few minutes, take a few deep breaths, and open your eyes. Once you're able to imagine a simple object in all its detail, you can move on to something more difficult.

Step Two: Visualizing a changing image

It's usually simple to imagine an object that's static. All we have to do is look at it. But in this next step, we're going to be more creative and learn to change our image. This is where creativity comes in. Let's stay with the flower, except now you're going to imagine that it's rotating and that you're seeing it from all sides. As it turns, see the differences in texture and the slight variations in color. Now change the color. If the flower was white, imagine it turning orange. Change the shape. If it was round, see it beginning to elongate and take on a totally different appearance. Imagine the new flower for a few minutes, take a few deep breaths, and open your eyes.

Step Three: Visualizing movement

The next step in learning to visualize is to imagine an entire scene and also add movement. For example, close your eyes and imagine yourself flying over an entire field of flowers and beautiful scenery, looking down at trees, a winding river, animals moving through the forest, and meadows filled with those colorful flowers. As you're flying, look down at the tops of the trees and see birds fluttering through the branches. Look closer and see the shapes of the trees and the texture of the bark. Now swoop down and get close to the water rushing along the banks of the river. Feel the wind and the spray of water against your face as the river takes sudden twists and turns. Finally, float down into a meadow and lay on the soft grass surrounded by flowers, looking at a blue sky and wisps of clouds slowly passing above you. Take a few deep breaths and open your eyes.

These are just three exercises that should strengthen your ability to visualize. Remember, visualization is all about using your senses to create images in your mind, not about using your mind to think about things analytically. As you practice visualization, you'll become much better at allowing your mind to evoke feelings and to observe even the smallest details. Eventually creative imaging will become as automatic as daydreaming.

The Five Elements of Guided Imagery

There are as many imaging exercises as there are people who imagine, so the type of image that works best for you depends on your personality, your experiences, and your preferences. In other words, for imaging to work well, it needs to fit you as an individual. But just as there are rules and guidelines for meditation, there are guidelines for imaging.

1. **Make comfort a priority.** Because guided imagery is basically a relaxation technique, it works best when you're completely comfortable. The smallest tension or discomfort caused by poor posture, hot or cold room temperature, binding clothes, etc. will affect concentration and disrupt your image.

2. **Use familiar images that you know will help you relax.** Effective images originate from your past, and trigger strong memories. However, make sure those memories are good ones. Don't use an image of the beach, for example, if you hate sand and bright sun. On the other hand, if mountains or a forest are what give you the greatest pleasure and help you relax, then use those as your mental image. If another image keeps cropping up in your mind, then that particular image may be stronger and more effective than the one you thought was perfect. You'll know when you've find the perfect image when it evokes relaxation almost immediately.

3. **Always begin with smooth and even breathing.** Like meditation, the key to effective imaging is proper breathing, which makes it easier for your mind and body to become more relaxed. Before starting an imaging exercise, spend a few moments breathing smoothly and evenly, and really concentrate on feeling your body relax and become tension-free.

4. **Make your images animated.** Memory experts use tricks to help people remember facts. One of those tricks is to make mental images animated. For example, if your image is one of you lying on a beach, make the water gently lap along the shore and warm, gentle breeze blow across your body. Dull, static images are never as powerful as ones that are colorful and dynamic.

5. **Choose images that are real and have meaning.** Most of us are pretty good at fantasizing, but unless we practice visualization, fantasies tend to be intermittent and fleeting. So the best images not only are ones that gives us pleasure, but they come from our own experiences because they're more vivid and are part of our long-term memory.

Imaging Exercises for Relaxation

The key to effective guided imagery is a strong ability to visualize. If you've practiced and mastered the three visualization exercises at the beginning of this chapter, you're ready to use guided imagery for relaxation and for self-healing. But as a final exercise to help enhance your inner vision to its fullest, try to visualize an entire set of different scenes, one right after another. So close your eyes and try to actually imagine the following scenes. Add your own if you like. The more you do this, the better you'll get at intensifying the images you visualize.

- A car speeding around a winding road.

- A gentle breeze passing through a stand of trees.

- The incoming tide lapping against a shoreline.

- A horse grazing along a green meadow.

- Children laughing as they run across the yard.

- The pitter patter of rain against a roof.

- Waves crashing against the shore.

- A field of golden wheat swaying in the breeze.

- Puffs of white clouds moving across the sky.

- Rays of the sun heating up your body.

- Someone's hands rubbing your back.

There are literally hundreds of examples of imaging exercises, each one as unique as the individual doing it. The following examples are two of the more popular ones I use in my stress management seminars. Use these with the idea that you'll take the basic outline, change it if you like, and incorporate your own personal image into it. Although you may want to use one of the exercises offered here, be aware of your own personal needs and desires in order for this stress management/self-healing tool to work for you. Remember, it's important for an image to fit the individual and not the other way around.

Imaging Exercise #1: A Tropical Beach

Sit or lie down in a comfortable position, close your eyes, and breathe slowly and evenly. Concentrate on your breaths, and feel the sensation of the air moving in and out of your nostrils. With each breath you take, your muscles become heavier and heavier, and the tension begins to melt away. Now imagine that you're lying on a warm, tropical beach, the rays of the sun covering you from head to toe in its warm glow. Above you, there's a beautiful blue sky, and around you are colorful flowers and green plants swaying in a gentle breeze.

Continue to breathe slowly and deeply as you feel the sun's rays penetrate your body and make you feel even more relaxed. The sand beneath you feels warm and soothing as it caresses your body. Your muscles begin to feel so warm that they are now limp; so limp that your entire body drifts deeper and deeper into a state of total relaxation. Each time you exhale, your muscles become more limp and your body becomes more relaxed. And as the rays of the sun bathe you in warm light, and a gentle breeze swirls around your body, imagine yourself completely at peace.

During this exercise, some people find it helpful to use a mantra every few breaths in order to strengthen the response and condition the brain to evoke relaxation. You might say to yourself, "I feel warm and relaxed," or you may just say the word "relax" over and over. Continue the exercise for ten minutes, then open your eyes and stay relaxed for another minute or so.

Imaging Exercise #2: A Blue Lagoon

Begin this exercise as you did exercise #1, but this time visualize yourself floating in a turquoise blue lagoon surrounded by palm trees and beautiful tropical flowers. Above you, the sky is perfectly blue with wisps of small white clouds drifting across. A soft, tropical breeze sweeps across your body as you float effortlessly in the water, which envelops you and makes your muscles feel smooth and relaxed. As you breathe evenly and deeply, the water begins to massage your legs, moves slowly up to your arms, and finally the rest of your body. The warm water now penetrates your muscles, making them feel like all the tension is melting away. You're now completely weightless, floating gently and are at one with the water. With each breath you take, the warm, soothing water lifts you slightly; and with each exhalation, you sink back down and more tension melts away.

Some individuals do this exercise while taking a warm bath because it helps the image become vivid and real. Just make sure that your head is propped up on a bath pillow to prevent it from slipping down into the water and ruining the exercise. Continue the exercise for ten minutes, then open your eyes and stay relaxed for another minute or so.

Guide Imagery for Motivation

There are times in everyone's life when they need a little motivation. Think back to the last time you wanted to start a diet or an exercise program. What's the first thing you did? You thought about it. You reflected on your goals and the obstacles you would have to overcome in order to achieve those goals. And then you thought about your success and how good your life would be once you realized that success. Visualizing your final goal, therefore, and the steps you need to take to get there, is a powerful way to motivate and keep you on track.

Let's take as an example your goal of bench-pressing 200 pounds. I'm only suggesting this because this is how I personally motivate myself when strength training. The important part of this exercise is to be confident and to believe in yourself and your ability to break barriers. By imagining yourself training, and successfully executing each step along the way, you'll gain more confidence in your abilities, and your mind will prepare your body for the activity itself. Here is an example of how you might use a five-minute guided imagery exercise for motivation and success.

1. Identify the goal you want to visualize—in this case bench-pressing 200 pounds.

2. Find a comfortable place to sit and relax. Eliminate distractions; turn off the phone, television, etc.

3. Close your eyes and breathe smoothly. Don't begin until you've freed your mind of any intruding thoughts.

4. Now imagine yourself in the gym. See yourself lying down on the bench looking up at the barbell. Feel yourself squeezing the bar and tensing your shoulders, forearms, and back as you ready yourself to lift the weight. Now visualize yourself taking a deep breath, lifting the bar off the rack, and lowering it to your chest. As it barely touches your chest, visualize yourself strong enough to lift the weight back up as you breathe out.

5. Take a few seconds to feel the pleasure and excitement of achieving this goal.

6. Rest for a few seconds and do it again.

The main point of this exercise is to program your mind to believe that you can accomplish your goal. A common mistake people make is to visualize unrealistic goals, which then destroy confidence and stifle progress. If your goal is to lift 200 pounds, don't visualize yourself lifting 200 pounds right away. Use mini-goals and gradually work your way up. In other words, if you lifted 175 pounds for the last three weeks, visualize yourself lifting 180 pounds this week. By changing your goals gradually, and visualizing continued success, you'll stay more focused and motivated.

Guided Imagery and Self-Healing

Visualization works so well because the images we create in our mind actually trigger physical responses in our body. Details such as texture, sight, sound, and smell, although created and imagined, are very real to the brain, which then uses those details to release hormones, regulate metabolism, slow heart rate and blood pressure, and boost immunity. The time we spend visualizing can be one of our most positive and life-changing experiences.

For those suffering with disease, the body is often regarded as the enemy. Negative feelings and attitudes are common during those trying times because we tend to start thinking of our body as a source of distress rather than a source of health and energy. We develop fears and anxieties that become worse and lead to a spiraling cycle of depression and hopelessness. And we give up on ourselves because we can't believe that the body responsible for the disease in the first place is able to fight it at the same time.

As we age and become sick more often, the mind accelerates the disease process through negative thoughts and perceptions, creating a cycle that is hard to break. Even younger people often give up when they succumb to disease because they don't accept nontraditional methods of healing as a viable option that can work when other treatments don't. Remember the power of the placebo effect discussed earlier. Creating positive beliefs through imaging can actually stimulate our immune system by helping us use the mind in a way that triggers a variety of disease fighting physiological responses.

The benefits of guided imagery result from positive expectations and attitudes toward illness. Together with traditional medical treatment, which should always be a principal source of therapy, imaging can have a tremendous effect on reversing the disease process while creating a mental environment that enhances the healing process.

Self-healing exercises are effective because we condition our mind-body connection to stifle stress reactions and trigger a stronger immune response, both of which enhance our body's ability to heal itself. These exercises also help maintain homeostasis by strengthening our neuro-endocrine-immune system, which aids our ability to resist disease in the first place. And finally, they condition our brain to respond to illness directly by altering the way in which our organ systems respond to a change in our physiology. So by using the power of visualization to help fight disease, we truly increase our ability to regain health and vitality.

Imaging Exercise for Self-Healing

Guided imagery for self-healing requires that you visualize the illness as vividly as you can and then imagine yourself conquering it. Here is an example of a general self-healing imaging exercise. Later, I'll discuss more specific imaging exercises used successfully by patients with various types of cancer.

Begin this exercise as you would any other imaging exercise—in a comfortable position, with your eyes closed, and with an even, rhythmic breathing pattern. Deepen your relaxation by breathing slowly and counting down from ten to one, one number for every exhalation. As you count, release more tension and allow your body to become heavier and more relaxed. Feel your body becoming more limp each time you exhale. Once you're relaxed, visualize the part of your body that's a source of illness. Try to see it as vividly as possible. If you're not sure what a specific organ or body part looks like, consult a medical guide beforehand. According to therapists, the more vivid, detailed, and accurate an image is, the better your chances are of using this technique successfully.

As you relax, and breathe slowly, see the organ or body part clearly in your mind. Watch the blood circulating through that organ, bringing with it oxygen and nutrients that enrich and heal, energize and invigorate. With every breath you take, visualize more and more warm, life-giving blood flowing into the organ or body part and removing toxic wastes and damaged cells. See the organ glow red with health and vitality, and picture yourself in perfect health with no sign of disease or illness. Continue this mental imaging for about twenty minutes before slowly opening your eyes and stretching.

Use this guided imagery as specifically as possible by visualizing the actual organ or body part. For example, if the stomach is the problem, you might want to visualize it being covered and repaired by new cells. Warm, healthy blood flows over the damaged area, bringing with it the new and healthy cells. As more and more life-giving blood washes over the damaged tissue, it becomes healthier and disease-free. Next, visualize yourself healthy and stress-free, completely free of illness.

Almost any illness or disease can be visualized this way with good success as long as you don't expect instant results. You have to remember that mental imaging is a process of visualizing an eventual desired outcome, not an instant miracle cure. So, although it's important to have a positive image and actually see yourself becoming well, it's also important to realize that imaging is an ongoing process that mobilizes your immune system and moves you steadily toward the end result. Hoping for immediate results will only lead to anxiety and frustration. Therefore, for optimum results, always visualize not only the process of healing but the positive and successful end result as well.

Fighting Cancer with Imaging

Although doctors have suspected for some time that the mind plays a key role in the development of cancer, it wasn't until the late twentieth century that guided imagery was recognized as a promising supplemental treatment. One of the concerns was that patients would opt for imagery rather than traditional treatment. But as more studies were done, researchers found that guided imagery not only reduced the effects of the disease but reduced the side effects of treatment. By the 1990s, guided imagery was used in many hospitals; and even the American Cancer Society had accepted it as a useful adjunct to regular treatment.

What finally convinced many doctors to change their thinking was a group of studies that showed guided imagery actually boosted immune function. In a 2008 study, patients with breast cancer either received guided imagery intervention or standard care. Four weeks after surgery, the group receiving guided imagery showed significantly higher NK cell activity against cancer cells.[24] A year later, another study found that guided imagery stimulated T cells and increased anticancer defenses during and after chemotherapy and radiation.[25] And in a recent 2011 study at the University of Texas M.D. Anderson Cancer Center in Houston, researchers showed that men with prostate cancer who used guided imagery had significantly higher NK cell cytotoxicity and other tumor fighting responses compared with controls.[26]

While these studies and others have clearly shown the positive effects of guided imagery, this complementary treatment should be a way to enhance the healing process and never a substitute for traditional therapy. Since cancer invades organs and causes a breakdown in the body's immune response, anything that boosts that response will have a destructive effect on cancer cells. In order to maximize the effect of guided imagery in ridding the body of cancer, you should follow three important rules:

1. **Condition yourself to relax.** Guided imagery is difficult unless your mind and body are completely at rest. Once you've learned to trigger the relaxation response, the neuro-endocrine-immune system will respond as well. Practicing meditation techniques before you begin visualization will help you achieve a much better outcome.

2. **Know what your cancer looks like.** You can't visualize something if you don't know what you're visualizing. Look up the type of cancer you have and study it. Make it more real and personal so that you're able to see it in your mind when it's being destroyed. To make the exercise even more effective, visualize the cancer inside the specific organ that's being attacked.

3. **Visualize positive results.** By now you know how powerful negative mental images can be. What's the point of using guided imagery if you visualize cancer cells not being destroyed? So it's critical for success to end each session with cancer losing the battle and being wiped out. The more you view positive results, the more your mind-body connection will become conditioned to respond in a more forceful way.

Each guided imagery session must begin with proper breathing and a relaxation exercise such as meditation or progressive muscle relaxation. Conditioning your body to relax is critical, because if you don't become deeply relaxed and tension-free during imagery, the healing process will not be as effective.

Once you're totally relaxed, begin visualizing the specific cancer in a way that's most powerful to you (a mass of tissue, a blob with spiked fingers or jagged teeth, for example), or visualize the cancer exactly as you've seen it in a book. Think of these cancer cells as weak and helpless, and easily destroyed by your body's immune system. Now visualize the treatment you're undergoing as strong and powerful. Radiation, for instance, may be seen as bursts of light energy, shattering the cells into a million pieces, which are then swallowed up by thousands of hungry, white blood cells. Chemotherapy can be visualized as a bright chemical that poisons the cancer cells but leaves the normal cells alone.

To be most effective, imaging exercises should be performed several times a day for at least fifteen minutes at a time. It's the repetition that leads to mind-body conditioning. It's also critical to visualize the cancer responding to the treatment and the healthy cells not affected and becoming healthier. Finally, never focus on the negative aspects of the cancer, but rather on the positive healing process so that you allow the mind-body connection to maximize the immune response.

The Best Self-Healing Images for Cancer

Researchers found something remarkable when they looked at scans of cancer patients who used strong, positive, and familiar images as opposed to patients who used weak and unfamiliar images during their treatment. The first set of patients became conditioned to respond much more quickly to the imaging exercise, and they were much better at triggering the body's immune system. This discovery proved that something as simple as an image can trigger a powerful self-healing response, as long as the image is seen as more powerful than the disease itself.

As described by the late O. Carl Simonton, MD, an oncologist who pioneered the use of the mind-body connection in cancer treatment, specific images can be so effective in fighting cancer because they have the power to create a strong belief in recovery. Because the mind part of the mind-body connection is just as important when it comes to self-healing, it's essential to use strong and positive images that get the body into cancer attack mode. Dr. Simonton's research suggested that five elements create the most effective and powerful self-healing images.

1. **An overpowering treatment that destroys tumors.**
   Patients who are at their most vulnerable often view cancer as unstoppable and overpowering, which may be why their immune systems fail them. Instead, they need to visualize cancer as weak, and their treatment as powerful enough to destroy it. To make that image most effective, the cancer should be a neutral color like gray or light brown and the treatment should be a distinctive, bright color like red or yellow, which makes it easier to visualize. Children, who are usually good at visualizing, could start off by drawing pictures of the cancer using different colored crayons to make the distinction between good and bad cells.

2. **Soft and fragile cancer cells.** Continuing the idea that cancer cells are not overpowering, patients need to condition the mind to see those cells as weak and helpless in the face of strong treatment. According to researchers, you must never use the colors black, red, or orange for cancer cells because these colors trigger strong emotions. Always use those colors for the treatment.

3. **Normal healthy cells.** The problem with most treatments is that, in the process of destroying cancer cells, they also destroy many healthy cells as well. To help stimulate the body's ability to recover, it helps if patients visualize their normal cells as strong and healthy enough to withstand the onslaught of treatment. As the chemo or radiation is destroying the soft and fragile cancer cells, the normal healthy cells are repaired quickly and remain strong and vibrant.

4. **Aggressive NK cells.** When a person develops cancer, the immune system sends out special natural killer cells whose only job is to kill cancer cells. Because these NK cells are so important, patients need to visualize them as extremely aggressive, attacking the cancer like an army of soldiers that destroys everything in its path. Just as important, though, is to visualize the dead cells being flushed from the body so that nothing is left behind to threaten again. The most powerful images, according to researchers, are ones in which cancer cells are outnumbered and overwhelmed so that the brain is conditioned to see the body's defenses as stronger than the disease. They also found that using familiar images such as swords that slice the cancer tissue away are more effective.

5. **A successful and positive end result.** As everyone knows, having a positive attitude can bring about remarkably positive results. Cancer patients who are depressed and negative seem to have the worst

outcomes, despite the best treatments. So, even after the final treatment is over, it's critical for patients to visualize themselves as cancer-free, and winning the battle over their illness.

Guided imagery should never be the only treatment option. But recent studies clearly show that using imaging together with traditional therapy is more effective than traditional treatment alone. That's because the brain can easily be conditioned to trigger a strong immune response that stimulates the release of NK and white blood cells. The more you use these imaging exercises, especially if you follow the guidelines for creating powerful images, the more spontaneous and effective they become.

In the past decade, more physicians have been using guided imagery as a weapon in their overall arsenal against disease. They haven't abandoned traditional therapies, but they've come to realize that the mind-body connection is much more powerful than ever imagined, and that treating virtually any illness can be enhanced if we take advantage of the brain's remarkable ability to heal the body. As researchers learn more about how imaging affects health and immunity, the more common and more successful these techniques will become.

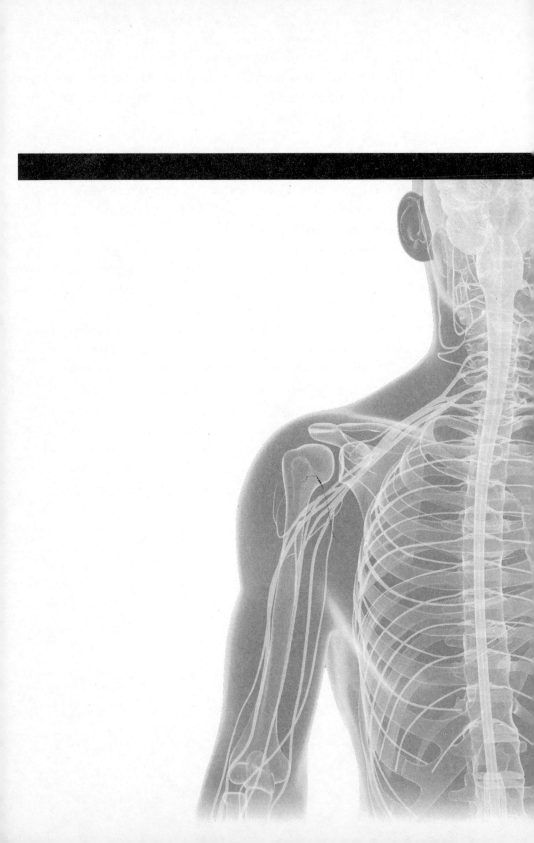

CHAPTER NINE

Relaxation Exercises and Techniques

Relax, You Are in Good Hands

As we saw in the previous chapters, relaxation techniques include a number of practices such as mediation and guided imagery. The goal of any technique is to consciously evoke the body's relaxation response and to use the unique power of the brain to reduce heart rate, lower blood pressure, and bring about feelings of calm and well-being. But in many cases, we need specific exercises and self-instructions that, when practiced enough, will condition the mind-body connection to respond in a way that triggers self-healing.

Because stress reactions are chemical events that affect immunity, they can trigger a host of physical and mental illnesses. So it's no accident that many patients visiting their doctors are doing so as a direct or indirect result of stress. What we've learned, though, is that perceptions and our ability to condition the brain can shape behavior and actually trigger positive immune responses. The link between the mind and body can be strengthened by specific relaxation exercises.

The fight-or-flight response, in which heart rate and breathing increase and blood vessels narrow, is a natural reaction to any type of stress. Over time, this natural response contributes to a range of health problems that will eventually lead to major disease. This is where relaxation exercises come in. By making them a normal part of our lives, they become a buffer that guards against the breakdown of homeostasis. According to the National Center for Complementary and Alternative Medicine (NCCAM), the key points about relaxation exercises are:

- Relaxation exercises are generally safe.

- Relaxation exercises consciously produce the body's natural relaxation response.

- Relaxation exercises often combine breathing and focused attention to calm the mind and the body. These are most effective when practiced regularly and combined with good nutrition, regular exercise, and a strong social support system.

- Most relaxation exercises can be self-taught and self-administered, and most require only brief instruction before they can be done without assistance.

- Relaxation exercises should not be used as a replacement for conventional care or to postpone seeing a doctor about a medical problem.

Relaxation exercises are the mainstay of any stress management program. In the past thirty years, research has focused primarily on illness and conditions in which stress appears to play a role either as the cause of the condition or as a factor that makes the condition worse. Currently, there is evidence that relaxation exercises are an effective part of an overall treatment plan for migraine headaches, pain, depression, asthma, heart disease and heart symptoms, high blood pressure, insomnia, and irritable bowel syndrome.

Meditation and guided imagery are two of the more popular and effective ways to reduce stress and boost immunity. This chapter describes how other types of relaxation exercises condition the mind and body to trigger the relaxation response.

No amount of attitude or behavior modification can totally replace relaxation as an effective tool for relieving the stress in our lives. Our goal should be to use everything available, including relaxation exercises, to keep organ systems healthy and in a state of constant readiness, should our homeostatic mechanisms fail us.

Progressive Muscle Relaxation (PMR)

Also called Jacobson's progressive relaxation or deep muscle relaxation, the principle behind progressive muscle relaxation (PMR) is that tension is incompatible with relaxation. We either do one or the other, but we cannot do both at the same time. If you spend much of your life in a state of tension, you have no idea what relaxed muscles are supposed to feel like. The technique developed by Edmund Jacobson, MD, a Chicago physician, trains us to differentiate between tensed and relaxed muscles. The underlying principle is brain conditioning; the end result is to familiarize us with what relaxation feels like compared with tension. As we do the exercise, we automatically block the signals that produce muscle tension and create a state that inhibits anxiety and negative stress reactions.

One of the best uses of PMR is to relieve insomnia. One recent study in women who were undergoing chemotherapy for breast cancer found that PMR significantly improved sleep quality and reduced fatigue by helping them relax their muscles and eliminate racing thoughts from their mind. For general insomnia, it may take a week or so to get good enough at it to induce sleep. But once mastered, PMR is one of the most effective ways to relax the muscles and bring about a sense of calm.

As effective as PMR is for reducing stress, anxiety, and insomnia, recent studies suggest that it may help with more serious disorders like schizophrenia. A systematic review of three controlled trials, for example, looked at the effectiveness of PMR in reducing psychological distress and anxiety in a total of 146 patients and found that PMR significantly decreased anxiety and increased subjective well-being.[27] New studies are being done to determine if PMR can reduce the need for antipsychotic and antidepressant drugs.

This simple technique consists of two things: conscious muscular tension followed immediately by relaxation so that the mind becomes acutely aware of the differences between the two. If we try to relax without first knowing the feeling of relaxed muscles, our body will not respond because our brain won't recognize tension as the stimulus it should be responding to. Tension-relaxation teaches us to discriminate between the two states so that our brain can instantly sense when and where tension occurs and to react to it in a natural and spontaneous way.

It's also important to be as comfortable as possible and to not have any distractions or disturbances during the exercise. After two or three weeks, you'll have conditioned your mind-body connection in a way that will make relaxing your muscles almost automatic. Even a small amount of tension will cause your brain to immediately recognize it and respond by triggering the relaxation response.

When you first begin PMR and are just conditioning the body to respond, always tense muscle groups separately. Once you master the technique, you can begin to relax various muscle groups together. For example, muscles in the hands and arms or the shoulders and neck can be combined so that relaxation is achieved by concentrating on whole muscle groups. Eventually, even tension can be eliminated since the relaxation response becomes a classic conditioned response.

When practicing PMR, the key element to success is being able to sense the change from being tense to being relaxed. If you can't do that, then go back to using maximum tension in order to condition your brain to recognize the difference between the two. The following are eight sets of standard PMR exercises, one for each muscle group. Remember to tense the individual muscles as much as possible for at least ten seconds before relaxing them. Repeat each muscle group three times before relaxing the entire body for ten to fifteen minutes. The greater the tension you exert, the more profound the feeling of relaxation will be. That profound change is what the brain will become conditioned to respond to.

PMR Set #1: Hands
Tension: Clench your fists as hard as you can for ten seconds.

Relaxation: Release your hands and let your fingers slowly uncurl.

PMR Set #2: Arms
Tension: Make a fist and contract your arms tightly for at least ten seconds.

Relaxation: Let your arms and fingers fall loosely at your sides and relax.

PMR Set #3: Legs
Tension: Without crossing your legs, bend your toes downward and contract your legs as hard as you can for at least ten seconds.

Relaxation: Let your feet and toes go loose and relax.

PMR Set #4: Abdomen
Tension: Contract your abdomen as much as possible for at least ten seconds.

Relaxation: Breathe out, lie perfectly still, and slowly relax your abdominal muscles.

PMR Set #5: Back

Tension: With only your head and buttocks touching the surface, arch your back and contract it for at least ten seconds.

Relaxation: Slowly lower your back and let it become loose and relaxed.

PMR Set #6: Shoulders

Tension: Shrug your shoulders as hard as you can for a full ten seconds.

Relaxation: Lower your shoulders slowly and let them become loose and relaxed.

PMR Set #7: Neck

Tension: Push your head backward against a pillow as hard as you can for a full ten seconds.

Relaxation: Let your head relax and just lie quietly and motionless.

PMR Set #8: Forehead/Face

Tension: Wrinkle your forehead and face as much as you can and hold it for a full ten seconds.

Relaxation: Release the forehead and facial muscles and let your face become completely relaxed.

When using PMR techniques, the following guidelines will make relaxation more effective and easier to learn.

- **Practice every day, even if it's only for a few minutes.** The more you practice, the stronger the conditioning becomes and the easier it will be to spontaneously relax. Early evenings are a good time to practice because the day's behind you and you'll be able to give your full attention to the technique. Right before bed is not as good since your mind is getting into sleep mode and brain conditioning is not as effective.

- **Wear loose, comfortable clothing.** The worst thing for relaxation is distraction, even if it's small. So, kick off your shoes, loosen your buttons, and remove any jewelry such as watches, bracelets, and necklaces.

- **Don't practice on a full stomach.** This can also be a distraction because digestion, especially during the hour after you've finished eating, will make you feel sluggish and full. And because much of your blood is being diverted toward your digestive system, you won't be as focused on the exercises as you should be.

- **Make the room quiet and comfortable.** Also a distraction, a room that's too noisy, not well ventilated, or too hot or too cold, will definitely lessen your ability to concentrate on the exercises.

- **Following tension, relax gradually.** If you relax abruptly, your brain won't recognize the subtle transition between complete tension and complete relaxation. For proper conditioning to occur, the relaxation part needs to be smooth and gradual, allowing a full ten seconds. Keep your eyes closed during the entire practice session and never cross your arms or legs.

PMR is one of the most effective relaxation techniques because it conditions the brain to recognize the difference between tensed and relaxed muscles. And once the brain does that, it will easily set into motion the chemical triggers that evoke the relaxation response. For most individuals, this can happen within a few weeks. With enough practice, you'll be able to induce muscle relaxation spontaneously without having to tense your muscles at all.

Autogenic Training (AT)

The degree to which our muscles are relaxed can be controlled by practicing a technique called autogenic training or AT, which is really a type of progressive muscle relaxation developed by Dr. Johannes Schultz in 1932. The objective is to induce deep muscle relaxation, not by tensing but by gradually releasing tension from various parts of the body, one part at a time. The muscles are trained, through specific autosuggestions and brain conditioning, to relax spontaneously in response to internal cues. These cues act as a signal for the mind-body connection to reverse course and switch off the fight-or-flight response.

Autogenic means originating within the body, so in essence you're self-treating without the use of medication, a therapist, or other outside source. In other words, you're telling your body what to do. And because it's quick and doesn't require any special equipment, you can practice it virtually anywhere. However, AT requires regular practice, so unless you're motivated to do this for several weeks in order to become proficient, AT may not be as effective as some other relaxation techniques. The disorders that have benefited most from AT are asthma, stress, anxiety, migraine headaches, high blood pressure, pain, fatigue, and insomnia. In fact, AT causes such deep relaxation that just fifteen minutes can make up for a poor night's sleep.

When doing AT, lie down or recline or sit in a comfortable chair with your back resting against a support. Beginners will find that lying down is most effective because it evokes the relaxation response the fastest. Once you learn a relaxation technique, any position can be equally effective and satisfying. Regardless of the position, comfort is critical. Pillows can be placed under the head, knees, and arms, or under the face, pelvis, and feet. The chair should be comfortable and have cushioned arms. Here are some rules to follow in autogenic training.

- **Get comfortable.** Just as you did for PMR, make comfort a priority. Take off your shoes, remove any jewelry, and loosen your belt. Make sure the room you're in is quiet and not too cold or too hot.

- **Pace yourself.** Speaking in a low, soft, even, and rhythmic voice will induce relaxation.

- **Breathe slowly but naturally.** Review the breathing exercises in the chapter on meditation, and make sure that each breath is long, smooth, and gentle. As you breathe, focus on your muscles becoming loose and tension-free.

- **Use soft words to help you relax.** Using words like smooth, heavy, limp, and relax will condition your brain to associate those words with relaxation. When repeating words such as relax, say them slowly as you breathe out.

- **Once relaxed, stay that way for several minutes.** Don't jar yourself out of the calm feeling you've just put yourself in. The purpose of AT is getting into this relaxed state, so spend some time enjoying it.

Unless the body is totally comfortable, relaxation is possible but won't be as effective. Therefore, body position and comfort are the principal starting points when beginning an exercise. Soft music can help you relax because you'll concentrate on the music and forget about other distractions. When listening to music, however, make sure that it's not too loud and never too harsh. Soft, classical music, such as that by Handel (Largo), Bach (Air on G String), Saint-Saens (The Swan), Barber (Adagio for Strings), is ideal for relaxation.

Autogenic Instructions

Autogenic training consists of six standard exercises that make the body feel warm and relaxed. After using these instructions several times, you'll know them by heart and be able to use them automatically whenever you feel tense. You may even want to shorten the self-instructions after becoming adept at bringing on relaxation. As you begin to condition yourself, you'll notice that relaxation will come more quickly and with much less effort each time. With enough practice, you'll be able to relax your entire body within a minute or so of starting an exercise.

Learning AT is simple because the mind is easily conditioned to respond to suggestions, especially if you practice on a regular basis. As a beginner, you should follow the six steps exactly, one step at a time, so that your mind-body connection will recognize the cues you're giving it. It's also important to practice at the same time each day until you become more proficient. Spend some time practicing the steps, and don't go on to the next step until you've mastered the previous one. When you reach step six, you'll have conditioned the mind-body connection in a way that will bring about remarkable well-being. But before you begin AT, you must first learn how to cancel or undo the changes that take place in your body and that last as long as you're in the autogenic state. The steps in AT are:

Learning to cancel: When you end an autogenic session, cancel it by stretching and saying softly, "**Arms firm, breathe deeply, open eyes.**" Make sure you don't open your eyes until you've relaxed your arm muscles again; otherwise your arms may continue to feel heavy for a while. Don't go on to step one until you've practiced canceling.

Step One: Inducing heaviness. The first step in AT is to make both your arms feel heavy. As you breathe deeply and smoothly, say to yourself, "**My right arm is very heavy.**" Repeat this six times and then say, "**I am completely calm.**" Do the same for the left arm. When you finish, cancel by saying, "**Arms firm . . . breathe deeply . . . open eyes.**" Unless you actually feel your arms becoming very heavy, don't go on to the next step. Instead, spend some time practicing this exercise until you can actually feel yourself inducing heaviness.

Step Two: Inducing warmth. This step relaxes blood vessels and increases blood flow. Induce warmth by saying, **"My right arm is very heavy."** (six times); **"I am completely calm."** (once); **"My right arm is very warm."** (six times); **"I am completely calm."** (once); **"My left arm is very heavy."** (six times); **"I am completely calm."** (once); **"My left arm is very warm."** (six times); **"I am completely calm."** (once). Repeat this sequence two or three times. Once you begin to feel warmth, you know that your body is producing physical changes and that this step is working. At the end, cancel by saying, **"Arms firm . . . breathe deeply . . . open eyes."**

Step Three: Heart practice. Once you're completely relaxed as a result of heaviness and warmth, your entire cardiovascular system benefits because your blood vessels have dilated and more oxygen is rushing through your heart. So now the full sequence would be, **"My right arm is very heavy."** (six times); **"I am completely calm."** (once); **"My right arm is very warm."** (six times); **"I am completely calm."** (once); **"My left arm is very heavy."** (six times); **"I am completely calm."** (once); **"My left arm is very warm."** (six times); **"I am completely calm."** (once); **"My heart beats calmly."** (six times); **"I am completely calm."** (once). Repeat the sequence two or three times and then cancel by saying, **"Arms firm . . . breathe deeply . . . open eyes."**

Step Four: Breathing practice. Breathing is a natural progression because by the time you get to this point, you're completely relaxed and your breaths are smooth and regular. Try not to control your breathing; allow it to happen on its own. The full sequence now becomes, **"My right arm is very heavy."** (six times); **"I am completely**

calm." (once); "**My right arm is very warm.**" (six times);"I am completely calm." (once); "**My left arm is very heavy.**" (six times); "**I am completely calm.**" (once); "**My left arm is very warm.**" (six times); "I am completely calm." (once); "**My heart beats calmly.**" (six times); "I am completely calm." (once); "**My breathing is calm and regular.**" (six times); "**I am completely calm.**" (once). Repeat the sequence two or three times and then cancel by saying, "**Arms firm . . . breathe deeply . . . open eyes.**"

Step Five: Abdominal practice. Once you've learned to get your arms and chest to relax, your heart to beat calmly, and your breathing to be smooth and regular, you can proceed to your abdomen. This can be a little tricky because sometimes the abdomen is tense and doesn't want to relax. This next sequence would be, "**My right arm is very heavy.**" (six times); "**I am completely calm.**" (once); "**My right arm is very warm.**" (six times); "**I am completely calm.**" (once); "**My left arm is very heavy.**" (six times); "**I am completely calm.**" (once); "**My left arm is very warm.**" (six times); "**I am completely calm.**" (once); "**My heart beats calmly.**" (six times); "**I am completely calm.**" (once); "**My breathing is calm and regular.**" (six times); "**I am completely calm.**" (once); "**My abdomen is warm and soft.**" (six times); "**I am completely calm.**" (once). Repeat the sequence two or three times and then cancel by saying, "**Arms firm . . . breathe deeply . . . open eyes.**"

Step Six: Head practice. The final step is proceeding to the head, specifically the forehead, which should feel cool. Coolness in the forehead is an indication of relaxation, so this last step is a good way to finish the exercise. The final sequence should be, "**My right arm is very heavy.**" (six times); "**I am completely calm.**" (once); "**My right arm is very warm.**" (six times); "**I am completely calm.**" (once); "**My left arm is very heavy.**" (six times); "**I am completely**

calm." (once); **"My left arm is very warm."** (six times); "I am completely calm." (once); **"My heart beats calmly."** (six times); "I am completely calm." (once); **"My breathing is calm and regular."** (six times); "I am completely calm." (once); **"My abdomen is warm and soft."** (six times); "I am completely calm." (once); **"My forehead is pleasantly cool."** (six times); "I am completely calm." (once). Repeat the sequence two or three times and then cancel by saying, **"Arms firm . . . breathe deeply . . . open eyes."**

Self-Hypnosis As a Relaxation Technique

Unlike hypnosis, in which a therapist puts you into a psychological state of heightened focus and concentration, self-hypnosis or autosuggestion is a way to relax your body and drive out negative thoughts by giving it simple instructions. Similar to autogenic training, self-hypnosis can be a powerful method to achieve very deep relaxation. The three steps involved are: 1) finding a quiet and comfortable space, 2) relaxing your body through deep and rhythmic breathing, and 3) deepening the relaxation through specific words that act as triggers. In the example below, I have a script that I use in my seminars that you can follow (don't say the words out loud), and which should make your session last about fifteen minutes.

I'm falling into a relaxed state; I'm breathing deeply, slowly, and smoothly . . . deeply, slowly, and smoothly. As I breathe, I'm becoming more and more relaxed . . . relaxed . . . relaxed. The toes on my feet are becoming numb; I feel a tingling sensation as the muscles in my toes become more relaxed and tension-free . . . relaxed and tension-free. They're getting more and more numb and heavy as I breathe . . . heavy and more numb. Now my toes are very heavy . . . heavy . . . heavy. The heavy, numb sensation is making my toes feel totally relaxed . . . relaxed . . . relaxed . . . more relaxed with each breath I take.

The numbness is beginning to creep up from my toes to my feet. My feet are beginning to tingle and are heavy and numb . . . heavy and numb. There's a warm sensation in my feet as if they were submerged in warm, refreshing water. As I breathe, I can feel my feet becoming numb and more relaxed. The muscles in both feet are becoming loose and soft . . . loose and soft; they feel warm, heavy, and relaxed . . . relaxed . . . relaxed . . . more relaxed with each breath I take. My feet are so warm and soft . . . warm and soft and relaxed . . . relaxed . . . relaxed . . . more relaxed with each breath I take.

I feel the warmth and numbness going to my calves as I breathe and relax . . . breathe and relax. My calves are beginning to get very heavy and numb . . . heavy and numb. They're getting soft and warm as tension leaves and muscles relax . . . relax . . . relax. With each breath I take, my calves are getting heavier . . . heavier . . . heavier . . . relaxed and numb . . . relaxed . . . relaxed . . . relaxed . . . more relaxed with each breath I take.

The numbness is moving from my calves to my thighs. My thighs are beginning to feel warm and soft . . . warm and soft . . . loose and relaxed . . . relaxed . . . relaxed. My thighs are getting numb and heavy . . . numb and heavy; there's a tingling sensation as they become numb and heavy . . . soft and relaxed . . . relaxed . . . relaxed. With each breath I take, my thighs are getting more relaxed and heavier . . . heavier . . . heavier. I feel the warmth and numbness creeping up my thighs and releasing tension. With each breath I take, my thighs feel more and more heavy and limp, limp and relaxed . . . relaxed . . . relaxed . . . more relaxed with each breath I take.

My fingers are beginning to tingle and get numb as the warmth creeps into them. They're becoming very soft and loose . . . soft and loose . . . warm and numb . . . numb . . . numb. I sense a numbness going from the tips of my fingers into my knuckles as I breath slowly and relax . . . relax . . . relax. The warmth and numbness is going into my wrists and my wrists are getting warmer and warmer . . . softer and softer. My hands are heavy and relaxed . . . relaxed . . . relaxed. With each breath I take, my hands are heavy and relaxed . . . relaxed . . . relaxed . . . more relaxed with each breath I take.

My arms are now beginning to get numb. The warmth is spreading from my hands into my arms, and I feel heaviness and warmth . . . heaviness and warmth. As I breathe, my arms are getting heavier and heavier . . . numb and relaxed . . . relaxed . . . relaxed. A tingling sensation is going up my arms and releasing tension; my muscles are beginning to relax . . . relax . . . relax. My arms are very heavy now and relaxed . . . relaxed . . . relaxed . . . more relaxed with each breath I take.

The numbness in my arms is creeping into my shoulders and my shoulders are now getting heavy and numb . . . heavy and numb. I can feel the warmth and heaviness loosening the muscles in my shoulders as they become relaxed . . . relaxed . . . relaxed . . . more relaxed with each breath I take. As I breathe, tension is flowing out of my shoulders and they now feel so warm and numb . . . warm and numb . . . heavy and relaxed . . . relaxed . . . relaxed . . . more relaxed with each breath I take.

Warmth is spreading from my shoulders into my chest and feels warmer and warmer . . . looser and looser. With each breath I take, my chest is more heavy and numb . . . heavy and numb . . . soft and relaxed . . . relaxed . . . relaxed. I can feel the muscles in my chest tingling and becoming numb and heavy . . . numb and heavy. As I breathe, tension is leaving. My chest is heavy and relaxed . . . relaxed . . . relaxed . . . more relaxed with each breath I take.

The numbness and warmth are traveling from my chest to my neck. My neck is becoming warm and numb . . . warm and numb. I can feel the tingling, numbing feeling in my neck as I breathe and relax . . . relax . . . relax. My neck is heavier and heavier . . . warmer and warmer . . . more relaxed with each breath I take. The tension is melting away from my neck and I feel so relaxed . . . relaxed . . . relaxed . . . more relaxed with each breath I take.

My body feels so warm and relaxed . . . relaxed . . . relaxed . . . heavy and numb . . . heavy and numb. My body is so heavy and relaxed that it's sinking into the chair. Tension is melting away; my body muscles are soft and relaxed . . . soft and relaxed . . . heavy and limp . . . heavy and limp. As I breathe, I feel soothing warmth washing over my entire body and I'm so totally relaxed . . . relaxed . . . relaxed . . . relaxed.

Self-hypnosis has been effective in relieving a variety of stress-related illnesses like hypertension, migraine headaches, digestive disorders, and ulcers. But even if we don't suffer from these kinds of disorders, using relaxation techniques such as self-hypnosis regularly can prevent a breakdown in immune function when we're chronically stressed.

After practicing this technique for a short while, relaxation becomes almost spontaneous. The body is geared toward responding to instructions from the mind, and we'll have conditioned ourselves to bring on the relaxation response just as we would any other natural, physiological reaction. Once we learn how our muscles should feel when we're relaxed, it becomes a matter of habit and conditioning to bring them into that relaxed state whenever we want to.

Biofeedback

The principle behind biofeedback is the mind's ability to influence body functions such as temperature, heart rate, blood pressure, blood flow, and muscle tension. Through training, one can induce deep relaxation by simply conditioning the body to follow conscious mental suggestions. Used together with other therapies to treat disorders such as chronic pain, stress-induced asthma, colitis, and insomnia, biofeedback has been shown to be even more effective than relaxation exercises in relieving symptoms of migraine headaches.

For centuries, practitioners of yoga and meditation have claimed that they can control body functions. Recent studies confirm this. The brain, because of its ability to become conditioned through repetition and autosuggestion, is a powerful force in controlling how the body's autonomic nervous system operates. Today, biofeedback is used not only in helping people relax and eliminate stress and anxiety but as part of cancer therapy, to relieve pain, reduce the effects of chemotherapy, restore bodily functions, and help boost immunity.

Biofeedback is noninvasive and is typically done with monitoring instruments controlled by a certified professional. A sound or light serves as a continuous feedback signal that monitors a specific body function and lets one focus on what the activity feels like. The simple, battery-powered home devices have not been found to be as reliable.

Results of biofeedback vary depending on one's ability to concentrate on physiological functions such as heart rate and muscle tension. As the process is repeated, the individual begins to sense changes and learns—much as in tension-relaxation exercises—what it takes to evoke a specific body response. With biofeedback instruments, there are five ways to measure body functions.

1. **Electromyogram (EMG):** This measures muscle tension, usually in the shoulders (trapezium), forehead, or jaw. Even slight electrical activity in the muscles is amplified and can be detected by a signal such as a tone or light. As the person becomes more aware of the electrical activity by associating it with the signal, he or she will respond by decreasing muscle tone and eliminating tension.

2. **Electrodermal Activity (EDA):** Also called Galvanic Skin Response or GSR, this device measures electrical conductance in the skin. Usually attached to your

hand or foot, this device emits a slight electrical signal through your skin. The greater your stress and anxiety levels are, the more active your sweat glands will be, and the greater the electrical conductance is. That's because gland activity is directly related to emotions. Lie detector tests often utilize this type of device to measure sweat gland activity.

3. **Thermal Biofeedback:** This device measures skin temperature, which decreases with tension and anxiety because blood flow is redirected away from the skin and toward muscles and internal glands.

4. **Finger Pulse:** This measurement reflects blood pressure, heart rate, and heart rate irregularities. By actually seeing and/or hearing the continuous monitoring of heart rate, for example, an individual begins to learn how to reduce the rate through breathing or another relaxation exercise or technique.

5. **Breathing Rate:** Irregular or rapid breathing can signal anxiety, tension, asthma, hyperventilation, or other respiratory problems. Like heart rate, breathing is monitored continually so that the individual can focus on what he or she needs to do to control tension and anxiety.

Sensate Focus Approach

The most common method of biofeedback employs monitoring instruments, but one can achieve the same results without having to be attached to instruments at all. This is the sensate focus approach, and the principle is similar to tension/relaxation. With any type of biofeedback, the mind senses or recognizes what the body is doing and then learns to change that action through mind conditioning. And just like using monitoring equipment to tell you what is happening, you can use your own sensations as a natural feedback instrument.

One of the first to use sensate focusing techniques was the team of Masters and Johnson, the famous sex therapists who developed a program to help their patients overcome sexual problems. In the program, patients learned to focus on feelings and sensations they were having during foreplay and intercourse. By focusing on specific sensations within erotic zones, trainees were able to form habits and condition themselves to eliminate sexual problems.

Sensate focusing for the purposes of feedback and relaxation works on the same principle. A person concentrates on a sensation in a particular region or part of the body and gradually learns what it feels like to change that sensation. The following suggestions will help you use this technique most effectively.

- **Make yourself comfortable.** Any tension, especially in the body part you're trying to focus on, will interfere with the sensation. It doesn't matter whether you sit or lie down as long as you ensure that nothing stifles your concentration.

- **Begin focusing on the body part that feels the worst.** For beginners, this is especially important. It's not easy to discern sensations that you've become accustomed to, or ones that are not very intense. By trying to feel the most intense sensations, you'll be more successful.

- **Once you've focused on the sensation, stay with it as long as you can.** This may not be easy at first, since your mind will tend to wander and not focus. As you progress, you'll be able to stretch your sensate focusing from thirty seconds to a minute and eventually to several minutes. The longer you can hold your concentration, the more conditioned your brain will become and the more focused you'll be.

- **Imagine the changes that occur.** As in guided imagery, your body is more apt to respond to strong mental images. Once you've focused on a particular sensation (tension in your back, stomach pain, heart rate, etc.) feel that body part changing as you imagine yourself becoming more relaxed.

We know that stress isn't something we can touch or see, but rather a physical response triggered by the way we perceive life and react to events and situations. To overcome that response, we need a strategy that focuses on both mind and body, that changes attitudes and behaviors, and helps bring our body back into a state of rest and balance. In the next chapter, we'll see how spirituality, prayer, and a wide range of complementary and alternative medicine approaches are being used to strengthen the mind-body connection and speed up the healing process.

CHAPTER TEN

Spirituality, Alternative Medicine, and Health

That's the Spirit

Based on current scientific research, there's no longer any doubt that spirituality in one's life can affect health and self-healing. But exactly what is it about spirituality with or without the power of prayer that helps us heal? Most researchers, who until now have dismissed that question as irrelevant to science, are beginning to study this phenomenon and are coming up with some fascinating and illuminating answers.

The National Institutes of Health have recently funded a group of US scientists to study the effects of prayer on the health of cancer patients. The focus of the investigation is to determine if prayer can actually improve health and stimulate healing. Patients, who are randomly recruited and whose cancer has not spread to other organs, organize one or two months following surgery and run a prayer group for twenty-four weeks in which they meditate and pray for intervention. At the end of the session, researchers determine how the patients who had prayed for healing compare with those who had not. If successful, other such studies will no doubt follow in an effort to discover how prayer helps us heal and what kinds of spiritual interventions work best for individual patients.

According to a major CBS News poll of 825 people, 80 percent of respondents believed that prayer or other spiritual practices speed up healing and 64 percent said they prayed for their own health and well-being.[28] It's not surprising that more and more physicians are incorporating prayer with standard treatment, the thinking being that if patients believe prayer will help them heal, then traditional therapy will be even more effective. Regardless of how it happens, treatment is all about healing; and if prayer, for whatever reason, boosts the immune system and helps one heal, then that's all that really matters.

Faith and the Mind-Body Connection

Since biblical times, people have believed that faith can heal. Just thumb through the Old and New Testaments and you'll find examples of prayer being used to treat illness and disease. Today, millions of people travel to places like Lourdes in France or Medjugorje in Bosnia-Herzegovina where believers claim to have witnessed apparitions, miracles, and spontaneous healings.

Regardless of denomination or sect, all religions have as a common denominator faith that a higher power can heal. Whether a person believes in God, Jesus, Buddha, Mohammed, or another spiritual entity doesn't matter when it comes to self-healing. It's the belief system that makes a difference; and the link between the mind, which perceives the healing as real, and the body's immune system, which is activated and strengthened by this belief system.

The question, then, is why are some people more likely to be healed by faith than others? And why does one person's cancer disappear completely, while someone else—who goes to the same church and believes in the same God—dies from his or her cancer? It seems unfair that the body responds so differently in people who practice the same faith. According to researchers, the answer lies in a person's attitude toward sickness, his or her will to live, and how the mind perceives the effect of faith and prayer on the healing process.

I've witnessed this myself. Two persons with similar cancers, thought to be terminal, are members of the same church. One dies within two years of beginning treatment while the other is in complete remission more than ten years later. I'd spoken to both individuals, saw them in church on a regular basis, and observed that the one who survived had a consistently positive outlook on life, an incredible will to live, and has centered her life around her faith and her spirituality. There was something extra in her life, and perhaps it was that something that had given her immune system the boost she needed to overcome her disease.

In many cases, the faith one has in a higher power and that entity's intervention in the healing process has a lot to do with the body's ability to boost immunity. Since belief is centered in the mind, and the mind is intimately connected with the body, it makes perfect sense that healing is often triggered in those who have a positive flow of energy between the two. But faith alone is often not enough; and that's where prayer comes to the rescue.

The Power of Prayer

From 1986 to 1992, researchers at Duke University Medical Center and Johns Hopkins University School of Medicine studied the effects of religion, meditation, and prayer on health. During those six years, the research teams studied nearly 4,000 individuals aged sixty-five and older and looked at their health problems and whether or not they prayed, read the Bible, or were involved in other spiritual endeavors. What they found was astonishing. The results of the study showed that people who rarely or never prayed were at a 50 percent greater risk of dying during those six years than people who prayed even once a month.[29]

Similar studies over the last few decades have added to a growing list of benefits showing that repetitive prayer increases blood flow, decreases blood pressure, relaxes muscles, improves brain function, and decreases the secretion of harmful stress hormones. In general, the conclusion seems to be that people who are religious or who pray tend to heal much faster and overcome their illnesses more effectively than those who are not spiritual and/or who do not pray.

Prayer has also been shown to alleviate the onset and development of mental disorders. A study reported in the *American Journal of Psychiatry* concluded that people suffering with depression recovered significantly faster if they had deep religious convictions. When the results were analyzed further, it was found that spiritual belief, not necessarily activity such as church attendance, was the important factor, and that the higher people scored on a spiritual conviction test, the faster they recovered from their mental illness.[30]

In another study, conducted at Sheffield Hallam University in England, researchers found that people who prayed were less likely to suffer from depression and other mental disorders than people who did not pray. In the study, 464 men and women aged eighteen to twenty-nine were questioned about their faith-related beliefs and then measured for their frequency of church attendance. In both men and women, the frequency of prayer was strongly associated with higher self-esteem and fewer symptoms of depression, anxiety, and other mental illnesses. According to the *British Journal of Health Psychology*, the reason for these findings is that those with personal spirituality have a sense of order, a positive perspective on life, a sense of control, and are more able to cope with stress.[31]

Using Prayer for Health and Self-Healing

Based on years of studies at major research centers that show a strong link between faith and healing, many doctors are convinced that patients who pray and depend on their faith to pull them through have a better chance of recovering than patients who don't. It may simply be a matter of positive thinking, or a belief that a higher power is somehow aiding in the healing process. Whatever it is, there's no longer any doubt that spirituality contributes to longevity.

Most people pray in their own words, asking for help during their treatment and recovery. Others need more structure. Centering prayer, practiced in the medieval church for centuries, is an ancient Judeo-Christian way of communicating that was lost until Trappist monks rediscovered it in the 1970s. The key element of centering prayer is the focus on one sacred word or phrase from scripture. A person may choose the word "mercy," for example, or any other word that indicates a divine presence, such as love, peace, grace, etc. A phrase such as "God, grant me peace" or "God, help me heal" is also effective. Centering prayer can also be used in conjunction with the imaging techniques discussed earlier. After doing an imaging exercise, one can spend a few minutes relaxing and using centering prayer as a good way to finish the session.

Passages from spiritual writings are also used in prayer, meditation, and healing services. Many people find it relaxing just to sit in a quite area and read a passage or two a day. Since many passages are only a few words long, it's especially helpful to reflect or meditate for a few moments on what you've read. In order to fully stimulate the mind-body connection through spiritual awareness, we should not just read the passage but also absorb it, understand it, and try to envision how the words will help the body heal.

The healing power of faith and prayer cannot be underestimated. Some experts say that spirituality is hardwired into our brains; others believe that the source of faith healing is the immune system's response to what the brain is telling it to do, and that people who truly believe they are being healed by faith are simply using the power of the mind-body connection as a trigger for self-healing. More and more physicians are using that connection to help their patients recover from illness, disease, and surgery. But regardless of what one believes, there's no longer any doubt that the brain is the most powerful organ of healing known to humankind. Knowing that and using the mind-body connection as an instrument of self-healing will help us stay healthy and disease-free throughout life.

Complementary and Alternative Medicine

Complementary and alternative medicine (CAM) is any health practice not currently an integral part of conventional healthcare. There are five major areas: 1) alternative medical systems, 2) mind-body interventions, 3) biologically based treatments, 4) manipulative and body-based methods, and 5) energy therapies. Within these five areas are countless individual therapies and treatments too numerous to list here. But in many of these therapies, the mind-body connection is intimately involved in the healing process, and the success of any treatment is dependent on how effectively the brain can stimulate the immune system.

For many people, the decision to use alternative treatments is often a last resort. Perhaps conventional treatments didn't work. Or maybe a patient just wants to make sure that his or her illness gets the full range of therapy to ensure success. Whatever the reason, it's important to approach alternative medicine carefully and to consider three important factors: (a) the safety and effectiveness of the therapy, (b) the expertise and qualifications of the provider, and (c) the quality of service. Under no circumstance should an individual begin alternative treatment unless he or she can address those three concerns.

Safety and Effectiveness

Safety, in general, means that the benefits outweigh the risks. A safe product or therapy is one that does no harm when used under defined conditions and in the manner intended. Effectiveness, on the other hand, is defined as the likelihood of benefit under typical conditions. Since there's usually less information available about the safety and effectiveness of alternative therapies than about conventional medical treatments, it's especially important for patients to be wise health consumers. In other words, ask questions, read articles, gather information about clinical trials, research findings, side effects, and potential dangers, and visit official medical websites to get as much information as you possibly can.

Expertise and Qualifications

Before selecting a practitioner/physician, most people at least like to know that he or she is qualified and competent to practice. A physician should be board-certified to practice medicine in his or her specialty. You wouldn't think of going to a doctor if you knew that there were a dozen malpractice lawsuits pending, would you? Likewise, before undergoing alternative medical treatment, always take a close look at the background, qualifications, and competence of any alternative healthcare practitioner.

Contact state or local regulatory agencies, medical boards, consumer advocate organizations, and other health regulatory agencies to find out about a specific practitioner's license, education, and accreditation, and whether there have been any complaints. Talk to others who have had experience with a potential practitioner. Most importantly, talk with the practitioner in person. If he or she is not easy to talk to, you won't feel comfortable as a patient. Ask about his or her qualifications, training, licensing, and certifications yourself. Once you've selected an alternative healthcare practitioner, the education process and dialogue between the two of you should become routine and ongoing.

Quality of Service

Quality of service is not necessarily related to the effectiveness or safety of a treatment or practice. An alternative healthcare practitioner may offer excellent service but a worthless treatment. Conversely, poor service may lessen the effectiveness of an otherwise effective therapy. Visit the office, clinic, or hospital. Take a good look at the surroundings and ask plenty of questions. How many patients are seen in a day or week? How much time is spent with each patient? What are the costs for the service delivered? Can the service be obtained only in one place or is travel required? The bottom line here is that alternative healthcare service must adhere to standards for medical safety and care.

One final note: always consult your primary healthcare provider about any alternative therapies or treatments you're thinking about undergoing. In some cases, herbal products and supplements may interfere with prescription medications you're already taking, making them less effective. In other cases, alternative treatments may actually make conventional treatment dangerous, and your physician may have to alter your entire treatment regimen. So, inform not only yourself but also your doctor about your plans to use any kind of alternative medicine. The following section includes descriptions of the most popular alternative health therapies used today.

Alternative Health Therapies

The term CAM refers to a group of diverse medical and healthcare systems, practices, and products that are not presently considered part of conventional medicine, i.e., medicine as practiced by holders of MD or DO (Doctor of Osteopathy) degrees and by allied professionals such as physical therapists, psychologists, and registered nurses. Some healthcare providers practice both CAM and conventional medicine.

The list of what's considered to be CAM changes continually, as those therapies that are proven to be safe and effective become adopted into conventional healthcare and as new approaches to healthcare emerge. The following are the most common alternative health therapies.

Acupuncture

Originating in China more than 2,000 years ago, acupuncture is one of the oldest and most common medical procedures in the world. The theory behind it is that the human body has more than 2,000 acupuncture points that connect with twelve main and eight secondary energy pathways called meridians. Inserting hair-thin needles into these points stimulates the central nervous system to release chemicals into the muscles, spinal cord, and brain. These chemicals either block pain (opioids such as endorphins, for example) or release other chemicals, which then act on the brain or stimulate physiological responses within the body's organ systems.

In 1996, the FDA approved acupuncture needles for use by licensed practitioners and requires manufacturers of acupuncture needles to label them for single use only. Still, complications may result from misuse of needles and from incompetent practitioners. To prevent problems, always check credentials and references. Increasingly, physicians have become familiar with acupuncture and may know of a certified practitioner; and as many as a third of all certified acupuncturists in the United States are medical doctors.

According to a National Institutes of Health (NIH) panel of scientists and researchers, clinical studies have shown that acupuncture, by itself or combined with conventional therapies, is often effective in treating pain, addiction, headaches, menstrual cramps, fibromyalgia, osteoarthritis, carpel tunnel syndrome, and asthma, and to assist in stroke rehabilitation.

The following are some conditions and disorders treated with acupuncture.

Acupuncture Treatments for Various Disorders

Chronic pain	Neck and back pain, migraines, strains, stomach pain
Cardiovascular	Angina, high blood pressure, palpitations
Digestive	Constipation, colitis, gastritis, hyperacidity, irritable bowel syndrome, indigestion
Emotional	Anxiety, depression, insomnia, overeating, smoking, substance abuse
Gynecological	PMS, menstrual symptoms, menopause symptoms
Musculoskeletal	Arthritis, carpal tunnel syndrome, cramping, joint pain, peripheral neuropathy, sciatica
Neurological	Bell's palsy, fibromyalgia, dizziness, numbness, neuralgia, neuropathy, restless leg syndrome, temporomandibular joint (TMJ) disorders
Respiratory	Allergies, asthma, bronchitis, sinusitis
Urogenital	Erectile dysfunction, incontinence, bladder spasms
Miscellaneous	Chronic fatigue, tinnitus, stress relief

Aromatherapy

Aromatherapy is the use of essential oils for relaxation and stress relief or to treat a variety of disorders such as colds, headaches, pain, circulatory problems, and indigestion. For centuries, people have been using oils in baths, as massages, or as aromatic vapors. In theory it works by stimulating the brain to release certain beneficial hormones while inhibiting others like cortisol. The most common essential oils are used as muscle relaxants, tonics, stimulants, immune system boosters, and to help repair damaged cells and tissues.

The term "essential oil" is used to describe the condensed or highly concentrated derivatives of a plant's flowers, seeds, stems, or bark. Sometimes a single drop of essential oil has the potency of an ounce of plant material. Today, the five most used essential oils are lavender, peppermint, eucalyptus, chamomile, and rosemary. There are many others on the market and you should become familiar with their safety and efficacy before using them.

Advocates of using essential oils say that they may not directly cure diseases, but there's no doubt that they affect ✓ mood and behavior. And by altering mood and behavior, they work on the mind-body connection in a way that can stimulate healing. New research has also shown that aromatic oils may help fight bacterial infections by slightly lowering blood pH and producing a more acidic environment that bacteria don't like. For this reason, it's also important not to overdo it. When it comes to aromatherapy, a little goes a long way.

Ayurvedic Medicine

Ayurvedic medicine (also called Ayurveda) is one of the world's oldest medical systems. Originating in India, it is a traditional system of healing arts that uses spices, herbs, vitamins, proteins, minerals, and metals. In the United States, Ayurvedic medicine is considered an alternative whole medical system. Many therapies used in Ayurvedic medicine are also used on their own as alternative therapies; for example, herbs, massage, and specialized diets. Because Ayurvedic products are not reviewed or approved by the FDA, there are a lot of scams on the market, so consumers need to be cautious when purchasing anything over the Internet. Recent investigations have shown the presence of heavy metal in as many as one-fifth of all Ayurvedic products sold in the United States.

Binaural Beats

Discovered in 1839 by a German scientist, H. W. Dove, binaural beats are brainstem responses to two tones played at different frequencies heard in opposite ears. The concept is remarkable in that, when each ear hears a different frequency through stereo headphones, the brain's superior olivary nucleus produces a third frequency—the binaural beat—that's perceived as a fluctuating rhythm. This specially generated rhythm induces relaxation, reduces pain, slows heart rate, improves sleep, enhances learning and creativity, and brings on a deep meditative state. Because each brain hemisphere has its own olivary nucleus, which receives signals from the ear and processes sounds, the binaural beats seem to synchronize the hemispheres and enhance brain function.

Binaural beats may have implications for medicine as well. Researchers in Thailand recently found that when patients underwent surgery requiring just local anesthesia, binaural beats made them feel less frightened and much less anxious and stressed. They also had lower blood pressure levels.[32] Physicians around the world are becoming more aware of this technique and are beginning to incorporate it into their practices.

Another benefit of binaural beats is that when the brain is in this altered state for as little as five minutes, it recalibrates and stabilizes the chemicals that are continually transported into and out of brain cells. When this happens, a person experiences less mental fatigue throughout the day and is much more alert and refreshed. To try this new technique, just get some headphones and download or buy a few binaural tapes. Each person will respond differently, so you may have to experiment a little to find the binaural beat that works for you.

Color and Light Therapy

When photoreceptors in the retina of the eye are stimulated, they trigger nerve impulses that travel to the brain's vision center. According to proponents of color/light therapy, by stimulating neurovisual pathways, we can decrease stress and tension, enhance learning, concentration, and memory, combat fatigue, mood swings, and depression, and improve mental and physical functions in general. It is increasingly well known that using high intensity white light can be very effective in treating Seasonal Affective Disorder (SAD).

For thousands of years, Chinese and Indian sages have claimed that certain colors have healing properties and that they can be used to treat a variety of illnesses. Greens and blues, for example, have a tendency to calm and soothe (thus, hospital walls are often painted with these colors), while reds and oranges can stimulate. Certain colors or color combinations are then used for therapy depending on the illness or the organ affected.

The use of colored lenses, which affect the optic nerve and stimulate a reaction, is growing in popularity, as is the use of crystals, which project color as light penetrates and passes through. Other uses include the color of carpeting, furniture, clothing, etc. The principle behind all this is that light and color affect the pituitary, which directs much of the endocrine system and controls body functions such as growth, metabolism, immunity, and sexual activity, and the pineal, which produces melatonin, the hormone that sets our biological clock and circadian rhythms. In essence, the specific frequency of each color can enhance our ability to heal, maintain proper levels of hormones, and keep the body in a state of natural harmony and balance.

Homeopathy

In 1790, after reading about a poison derived from a Peruvian bark known as cinchona, the plant that was used to treat malaria in those days, and the same substance from which quinine is derived, Dr. Samuel C. Hahnemann decided to perform an experiment on himself. It would be the first instance of what homeopaths refer to as "the proving of a remedy." He ingested the drug cinchona and carefully marked down his ensuing symptoms. The symptoms were indeed particularly similar to the symptoms of malaria. After experimenting with other drugs in the same manner, and then clinically practicing their results, Hahnemann concluded that the reason cinchona cured malaria was because it could produce similar symptoms to malaria if given to a healthy person. This is the basic premise of homeopathy: "Like Cures Like."

Homeopathy, then, is based on the Law of Similarities. It tries to stimulate recovery and self-healing by introducing a minute amount of a substance that causes similar symptoms. The substances are produced by homeopathic pharmacies in accordance with *Homeopathic Pharmacopoeia of the United States*, an official guide recognized by the FDA. Homeopathic medicines are derived from various plants, from minerals such as arsenic oxide or iron phosphate, and even from poisonous snake and insect venoms. All the substances are diluted until little of the original substance remains and the side effects are minimized, the theory being that the more diluted the substance is, the more potent and curative it will be.

According to scientific studies published in medical journals including the *Lancet*, homeopathy can be effective in treating a variety of illnesses such as asthma, arthritis, and migraines. Whether this is due to the treatment itself or because of a placebo effect or a combination of both is not known. But because homeopathic medicines are prepared from natural sources and diluted into extremely small quantities, they are safe and nontoxic. Like any other alternative therapy, however, patients need to learn all they can and consult with their physicians to ensure that homeopathic preparations will not interfere with other treatments.

Hydrotherapy

Also known as water therapy, hydrotherapy uses hot or cold water to relieve discomfort and promote physical well-being. Dating as far back as 4500 BC hydrotherapy promotes relaxation, reduces inflammation, lessens aches and pains, and promotes quick healing of muscle and joints. For pure relaxation, hot water or steam is used. To reduce inflammation and speed up recovery of muscles and joints, cold water is used. Alternating hot and cold water speeds up blood flow and affects the entire cardiovascular system. By using a combination of steam and essential oils that are inhaled, one can treat a variety of respiratory problems. Some common forms of hydrotherapy are whirlpools, saunas, hot tubs, water jets, steam treatments, soaking tubs, and showers.

Magnetobiology

Using magnets for healing is not new. In the third century BC, Aristotle wrote about the healing properties of magnets. The ancient Chinese, Indians, Arabs, Greeks, Hebrews, and Egyptians all used magnets for their healing properties. According to historians, Cleopatra used magnets to slow down the aging process. So, for at least two millennia, magnets have been considered a source of health and healing.

The principle behind magnetobiology is that magnets can alter electrical fields, and thus, it is theorized, increase the release of endorphins, restore pH balance, and increase blood flow and oxygen, which then speeds healing and restores the body's internal homeostatic mechanisms. Use of magnets for healing, specifically for relief of pain, arthritis, bursitis, back problems, muscles strains, and fibromyalgia is now anecdotally accepted in many countries including the United States. Magnetic wristbands, plasters, blankets, and mattresses are seen everywhere and sold by an increasing number of companies. This does not indicate that they are effective, only that they are relatively safe and readily available.

Mindfulness-Based Cognitive Therapy

In 1979, Jon Kabat-Zinn, PhD, a professor of molecular biology at the University of Massachusetts, developed an eight-week stress reduction program called Mindfulness-Based Stress Reduction (MBSR) to help treat patients at the UMass medical center. This highly successful program inspired Professors Zindel Segal and John Teasdale to develop Mindfulness-Based Cognitive Therapy (MBCT), which is now the treatment of choice for many health providers treating depression, anxiety, addiction, chronic pain, and stress.

The basis for MBCT is that an awareness of the body and the breath develops an awareness of the mind. By incorporating a specific meditative technique, learned over several weeks, patients learn to live in the present rather than contemplating the past or the future, and significantly enhance their quality of life. Mindfulness exercises help individuals recognize and accept what they cannot change, and gradually condition them to use their inner resources to heal themselves of emotional and physical disorders. MBCT is usually offered as an eight-week course, and practice at home is an important part of the training. Like any other therapy, it's not a quick fix; but once learned it can be used for the rest of one's life.

Music Therapy

Since ancient times, music and musical instruments have been used to soothe, relax, and influence health and well-being. The first official music therapy degree program in the world was founded at Michigan State University in 1944 as a way to use music to heal both physical and emotional disorders. Graduates of music therapy programs work in hospitals, clinics, day care centers, community health centers, psychiatric facilities, nursing homes, hospice programs, and in private practice. The primary therapeutic tool in all cases is music, which may include listening, singing, composition, and/or playing instruments.

Besides being an alternative treatment for illness, music therapy is used by healthy individuals for stress management, during labor and delivery, and for general maintenance of good health and a balanced life. In hospitals it is used along with medication to manage pain, by physical therapists to help rehabilitation, and by psychologists to counter anxiety and depression. Sessions are specifically tailored to meet the needs of the individual, taking into account likes and dislikes, culture, effect on behavior, emotional state, therapeutic goals, and state of physical health.

If you're considering music therapy, make sure the practitioner has completed extensive training in one of sixty-nine approved college music therapy curricula and has passed the national exam given by the Certification Board for Music Therapists. The exam assures that individuals have met accepted educational and clinical standards and are qualified to practice music therapy.

Naturopathy

During the nineteenth century, a "back to nature" movement started in response to the rapid social changes that accompanied the Industrial Revolution. Its main tenet was, and still is today, that illness and disease can be cured through the body's own natural healing and recuperative powers without the use of synthetic drugs or surgery. The doctor is simply there to help the process along. Naturopathic practitioners—who may be physicians, nurses, or physical and massage therapists—offer noninvasive treatments for a wide variety of disorders, but can also make use of lab tests, X-rays, and other exams to make diagnoses.

Naturopaths emphasize treatment of the whole person, which involves physical, spiritual, social, and emotional aspects. The cornerstone of all treatment, however, is diet and lifestyle; and the ultimate goal is prevention, so that disease does not arise in the first place. Practices and approaches include: dietetics, homeopathic medicines, herbs and botanicals, vitamin and mineral supplements, acupuncture, heat treatment, detoxifying enemas, fasting, physical therapy, biofeedback, and stress management.

According to scientific studies, some aspects of naturopathy work well while others have been found not to work or may cause side effects. Proper diet and nutrition, with an emphasis on fruits, vegetables, and whole grains, is widely accepted as standard, as is biofeedback, stress management, and acupuncture therapy. Other treatments such as herbal preparations, detoxifying enemas, and strict dietary restrictions may lead to serious health effects or they could interfere with conventional medical treatment. The greatest risk is using naturopathic remedies without consulting a physician, since a potentially life-threatening medical condition may go undiagnosed.

Orthomolecular Medicine

Linus Pauling, winner of two Nobel prizes, coined the word "orthomolecular" in 1968 to describe the use of natural products such as vitamins and other nutrients for health maintenance and in the treatment of disease. The key principle is that biochemical pathways and the concentration of enzymes, both of which affect the onset of disease when disrupted, can be corrected through the use of vitamins, amino acids, minerals, electrolytes, and fatty acids. In its early days, orthomolecular therapy included mega doses of nutrients.

Today, orthomolecular medicine, which still relies heavily on nutritional supplements, has expanded to include such areas as chelation therapy, hydrotherapy, heat therapy, phototherapy, electrotherapy, acupuncture, massage, biofeedback, and hypnotherapy. First and foremost, however, is nutrition.

Tai Chi

Originating in China as a martial art, tai chi is a mind-body practice that is also used in alternative medicine. It's sometimes referred to as "moving meditation," in which practitioners move their bodies slowly, gently, and with awareness, while breathing deeply. Tai chi incorporates the Chinese concepts of yin and yang (opposing forces within the body) and qi— sometimes pronounced "chee" (a vital energy or life force). Practicing tai chi is said to support a healthy balance of yin and yang, thereby aiding the flow of qi. There are many different styles, but all involve slow, relaxed, graceful movements, each flowing into the next. The body is in constant motion, and posture is important. Individuals practicing tai chi also concentrate, putting aside distracting thoughts, and breathing in a deep and relaxed, but focused manner. Some of the benefits include muscle strength, flexibility, improved balance, decreased pain and stiffness, and improved sleep.

Therapeutic Humor

Ever since Norman Cousins, author of the bestseller *Anatomy of an Illness*, claimed to have cured himself of ankylosing spondylitis, a progressive, debilitating, and degenerative disease of the joints, by watching hours of Marx Brothers and Three Stooges movies, laughter has been linked to the mind-body connection. In fact, humor and laughter have been associated with good health since biblical times. Proverbs 17:22 states that "A merry heart doeth good like medicine." The ancient Greeks built hospitals next to amphitheaters because they knew that patients would heal faster if they watched plays.

While in the hospital, Cousins was monitored during his bouts of laughter. Doctors found significant decreases in certain blood chemicals associated with illness and inflammation following the hours of laughing. Within months, Norman Cousins was living a normal, healthy life once again. His experience was published in the *New England Journal of Medicine*.

Numerous research studies have shown clearly that laughter increases heart rate, blood pressure, circulation, and oxygen intake, and has the same effects as aerobic exercise. At the same time, it lowers cortisol and boosts levels of white blood cells. William Fry, MD, of Stanford University claims that several minutes of intense laughter is equivalent to fifteen minutes on a stationary bike. For this reason, many hospitals and clinics are establishing humor facilities, which include humor rooms and areas where patients can watch funny movies and TV shows, or be entertained by comedians or clowns. The evidence seems compelling that a good belly laugh is also great medicine.

Therapeutic Touch

Healing touch is an alternative form of healing using the laying on of hands to treat illness. The principle behind it is that our bodies all have energy fields that become misaligned when the mind-body connection is disrupted and that these fields respond to touch. Practitioners claim that healing touch can help with pain, anxiety, stress, wound healing, hypertension, circulatory problems, cancer, arthritis, and diabetes. Parents know that hugging and touching their young children are critical for proper emotional development. Doctors know that the simple gesture of holding a patient's hand can make a world of difference in how that patient responds. So it's not a stretch for practitioners to believe that the laying on of hands—even if it's partially a placebo effect—can heal.

Today, more than 30,000 nurses and heathcare workers use therapeutic touch in one form or another. The world's first Touch Research Institute was founded at the University of Miami Medical School to study the effects of hands-on touch in the healing process.

Yoga

One of the six orthodox systems of Hindu philosophy, the goal of yoga is to attain higher consciousness and spiritual realization. It is usually practiced under the guidance of an advance practitioner who is trained in the spiritual disciplines of yoga. But besides the spiritual aspect of the discipline, yoga offers physical fitness through stretching and strengthening muscles, meditation to bring inner peace and physical as well as emotional health, stress management through proper breathing techniques and muscle relaxation, and a basic philosophy of life that emphasizes truthfulness, discipline, and spiritual fulfillment.

Yoga is often divided into eight stages: *yama* or restraint from vice, *niyama* or observance of purity and virtue, *asana* or posture, *pranayama* or breathing, *pratyahara* or withdrawal of senses, *dharana* or concentration, *dhyana* or meditation, and *samadhi* or internal peace. There are various traditions of yoga, but most have similar health benefits. Once considered exotic, yoga has become mainstream, with classes, online videos, and DVDs readily available. Numerous studies have demonstrated a clear physical and mental effect that improves circulation, blood pressure, lung capacity, and relaxation of muscles.

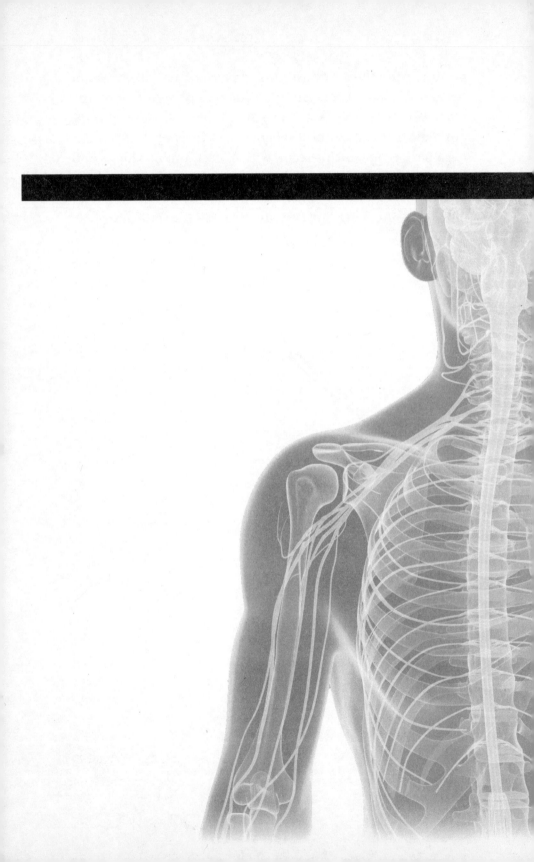

CHAPTER ELEVEN

The Mind-Body Connection in Children and Adolescents

We blame it on hormones, peer pressure, television, movies, and even the junk food they eat. But what transforms a youngster from a sweet, lovable child into a moody and disobedient teenager has more to do with brain development than once thought. Research shows that the preteen brain undergoes significant changes that influence both social interactions and impulsive activities associated with reckless behavior. It's during this critical time of life that the developing brain is affected and molded by traumatic events, emotional and/or physical abuse, alcohol, nicotine, and other substance use, relationships, and interactions with others.

Evidence based on MRIs and PET scans shows that nerve connections continue to sprout, develop, and grow during childhood and well into adolescence. This tells us that young brains are not yet mature enough to handle life stresses the way we expect them to. As a result, young people often have a difficult time organizing and planning, and they become impulsive and irresponsible. In short, they're responding to stress and their environment the only way their brains will allow them to.

According to Lynn Ponton, MD, a psychiatrist at the University of California–San Francisco and author of *The Romance of Risk: Why Teenagers Do the Things They Do,* "A big part of adolescence is learning to assess the risk in an activity. Part of the reason teenagers aren't good at risk-taking is that the brain is not fully developed." It's not really surprising, then, that behaviors such as smoking, drinking, and sexual promiscuity are a direct result of the adolescent brain not being wired in the same way as an adult brain.

Unlike adults, children and adolescents have a unique set of problems, and they perceive the world around them through a different set of lenses. In most cases it has little to do with the body and more to do with the mind. Because young minds are being bombarded from all directions and influenced by so many people in their lives, they are especially susceptible to stress reactions.

Because of their unique and sensitive time of life, it's important that we treat children and young people in a way that addresses their neurological differences. The mind-body connection may not be wired the way it will be eventually, but it exists nonetheless and it's an important part of a young person's overall health and well-being.

The Stress of Growing Up

Adults aren't the only ones suffering from stress or stress-related illnesses. In fact, childhood, and especially adolescence, can be a time of tremendous anxiety and emotional upheaval. Today, more than ever, young people are being diagnosed with depression, Attention Deficit Disorder (ADD), Attention Deficit Hyperactivity Disorder (ADHD), and a variety of other emotional problems associated with the stress in their lives. In the United States alone, a National Institute of Mental Health study has shown that as many as 6 percent of nine-to-seventeen-year-olds suffer from depression, with as many as 5 percent having major depression.

The reason children may *seem* less affected by stress than adults is that they're normally more resilient and less likely to succumb to stress reactions. Their immune systems are generally more responsive, helping them recover more quickly. And they tend to react to stressful situations with emotional and behavioral problems rather than physical symptoms.

According to experts, that's beginning to change. Both children and adolescents are experiencing unprecedented changes in society that are causing an epidemic of physical and mental health problems. To reverse this trend, we must first realize that young people are affected by the same mind-body connection as adults, and that healing will be most effective if they also learn to use their minds to heal their bodies.

The main categories of stress that affect children as they are growing up are life changes and events experienced by parents, life events experienced by families, and life events experienced by the child. The following chart lists the life events that cause the most significant stress in a child's life.

Parental Issues	Family Issues	Child's Issues
Death of a parent	Death of a sibling	Serious illness or disease
Separation or divorce	Birth of a sibling	Physical or sexual abuse
Substance abuse	Death of a family pet	Relationship problems
Unemployment	Relocation	Starting a new school
Imprisonment	Financial problems	Puberty
Major illness or disease	Separation from a parent	Change of friends
Remarriage	Vacation	Losing friends

Even though a child may not experience stressful life changes directly, he or she is still affected, sometimes more so than the parent or other family member. Divorce, separation, and death are traumatic events for children and adolescents, who feel confused and betrayed and sometimes blame themselves. Parents and caregivers need to recognize signs and symptoms of stress and intervene before it manifests as serious physical or mental health disorders.

Warning Signs and Symptoms

Children are not little adults, so the warning signs of childhood stress are often different from those in adults. But though children may experience unique symptoms at different stages of life, symptoms may overlap and, therefore, parents and caregivers should be on the lookout for any sign that may signal stress. Small, seemingly insignificant signs, especially if they are attributed to rebellious or normal childhood misbehavior, are sometimes overlooked. We shouldn't assume that a sudden change in behavior is nothing more than a passing phase.

The ages between six and twelve are a time of rapid brain growth, especially in the areas of language and understanding spatial relations. The age of twelve seems to mark the end of the critical period for learning languages. As children grow from preteens to teenagers, nerve networks increase at an astonishing rate. Every area of the brain is developing and maturing as quickly as the body but, according to new research, the part that recognizes and tempers reckless behavior does not fully develop until about the age of twenty-five. A young teenager's gray matter waxes and wanes at different times during development, with a rapid growth spurt in the planning, impulse control, and reasoning part of the brain just prior to puberty.

Because the brain is in a growth mode and is not completely mature, a young person may often have a difficult time planning, organizing, sleeping, handling stress, and coping with sudden changes in his or her life. Reactions to stress range from mild to severe and can create conflicts for the entire family. The following table identifies some of the main warning signs and symptoms exhibited by children at various stages of life:

Ages Six to Ten	Ages Eleven to Fourteen	Ages Fifteen to Eighteen
Bedwetting	Depression	Withdrawal
Excessive crying	Disinterest in school	Unusual loss of interest
Sudden thumb sucking	Unexplained poor grades	Loss of appetite
Unexplained fears	Aggression or violence	Sudden physical problems
Loss of appetite	Withdrawal	Personality change
Nightmares or insomnia	Inability to concentrate	Relationship problems
Stomach pains or nausea	Regressive behavior	Lowered self-esteem

At the youngest ages, children often act out or react because they're not yet able to communicate their feelings in a mature and constructive way. They may get frustrated or angry at something that older children can deal with more easily, so they lash out or they internalize, which then leads to issues like crying, thumb sucking, stuttering, bedwetting, or physical problems. Preteens have the added stress of puberty, emotional upheavals, social interactions, peer pressure, and physical changes. Girls at this age are especially vulnerable. The good news is that children at this age are still willing to communicate. Parents and teachers shouldn't pass up the opportunity to help them open up.

Teenagers, with hormones raging, bodies developing, and emotions in high gear, have an entirely different set of issues. They live in a world between childhood and adulthood and need more help in coping with stress than ever before. Parents need to be on the lookout for extreme moodiness, depression, or dangerous risk-taking, and not just assume it's part of normal teenage behavior. When asked to name the things that caused them the most stress, teenagers listed death of a parent or other family member as number one, followed by divorce, failure in school, parent losing a job, and romantic breakup.

It's natural for all children to experience some stress in their lives. But if symptoms of stress reactions persist for a long period of time, it may be an indication of a deeper root cause that needs to be identified and treated before the symptoms get worse. Sometimes talking about it will get at the core of the problem; often a professional needs to get involved. Parents should never take the position that kids will be kids and that they'll get over whatever it is that's going on with them.

Effects of Toxic Stress on Brain Development

The ability to manage stress is controlled by brain circuits and hormone systems that are activated early in life. When a child feels threatened, hormones are released that circulate throughout the body. Prolonged exposure to stress hormones can impact the mind-body connection and impair functioning in a variety of ways.

- Toxic stress can impair the connection of brain circuits and, in the extreme, result in the development of a smaller brain.

- Brain circuits are especially vulnerable as they develop during early childhood. Toxic stress can disrupt the development of these circuits. This can cause an individual to develop a low threshold for stress, thereby becoming overly reactive to adverse experiences throughout life.

- High levels of stress hormones, including cortisol, can suppress the body's immune response, which can leave an individual vulnerable to a variety of infections and chronic health problems.

- Sustained high levels of cortisol can damage the hippocampus, an area of the brain responsible for learning and memory. These cognitive deficits can continue into adulthood.

Research findings have shown that childhood stress can affect the mind-body connection in a way that impacts adult health. The Adverse Childhood Experiences (ACE) Study has demonstrated a link between specific violence–related stressors, including child abuse, neglect, and repeated exposure to intimate partner violence (IPV), and risky behaviors and health problems in adulthood. The study also provides strong evidence that being exposed to certain childhood experiences, including being subjected to abuse or neglect or witnessing intimate partner violence, can lead to a wide array of negative behaviors and poor health outcomes. In addition, the ACE Study has found associations between experiencing ACE and two violent outcomes: suicide attempts and the risk of perpetrating or experiencing IPV—specifically, the more adverse childhood experiences someone had, the more likely it was that he or she would attempt suicide and/or be the perpetrator or victim of intimate partner violence.

The Teenage Brain and the Mind-Body Connection

One of the ways that scientists have searched for the causes of mental illness is by studying the development of the brain from birth to adulthood. What they discovered is that striking changes take place during the teen years, in particular that the brain doesn't look like that of an adult until a person reaches his or her early twenties. This helps explain a puzzling contradiction of adolescence: young people at this age are at their peak of physical health, strength, and mental capacity, and yet, for some, this can be a hazardous age.

Mortality rates jump between early and late adolescence, rates of death by injury between ages fifteen to nineteen are about six times that of the rate between ages ten and fourteen, crime rates are highest among young males, and rates of alcohol and other drug abuse are high relative to other ages. These behaviors are all shaped by genes, childhood experience, and the environment in which a young person lives. Adding to this complex picture is that all these factors act in the context of a brain and a mind-body connection that is growing and changing, with its own impact on behavior.

A clue to the degree of change taking place in the teen brain came from brain scans of children as they grew from early childhood through age twenty. The scans revealed unexpectedly late changes in the volume of gray matter, which forms the thin, folding outer layer or cortex of the brain. The cortex is where the processes of thought and memory are based. Over the course of childhood, the volume of gray matter in the cortex increases and then declines.

The assumption for many years had been that the volume of gray matter was highest in very early childhood, and gradually fell as a child grew. The more recent scans, however, revealed that the high point of the volume of gray matter occurs during early adolescence. The scans also suggest that different parts of the cortex mature at different rates. Areas involved in more basic functions mature first, for example, those involved in the processing of information from the senses and in controlling movement. The parts of the brain responsible for controlling impulses and planning ahead—the hallmarks of adult behavior—are among the last to mature.

New research is showing that connections between different parts of the brain increase throughout childhood and well into adulthood. As the brain develops, the fibers connecting nerve cells are wrapped in a protein that greatly increases the speed with which they can transmit impulses from cell to cell. The resulting increase in connectivity—a little like providing a growing city with a fast, integrated communication system—shapes how well different parts of the brain work in tandem. The extent of connectivity is related to growth in intellectual capacities such as memory and reading ability.

The brain circuitry involved in emotional responses also changes during the teen years. The responses of teens to emotionally loaded images and situations, for example, are heightened relative to younger children and adults. The brain changes underlying these patterns involve brain centers and signaling molecules that are part of the reward system with which the brain motivates behavior. These age-related changes shape how much different parts of the brain are activated in response to experience, and in terms of behavior and the urgency and intensity of emotional reactions.

Enormous hormonal changes take place during adolescence. Reproductive hormones shape not only sex-related growth and behavior, but overall social behavior. Hormone systems involved in the brain's response to stress are also changing during the teens. As with reproductive hormones, stress hormones can have complex effects on the brain and, as a result, behavior.

In terms of sheer intellectual power, the capacity of a person to learn will never be greater than during adolescence. At the same time, behavioral tests, sometimes combined with functional brain imaging, suggest differences in how adolescents and adults carry out mental tasks. Adolescents and adults seem to engage different parts of the brain differently during tests requiring calculation and impulse control or in reaction to emotional content.

Adolescent brain-based changes in the regulation of sleep contribute to teens' tendency to stay up late at night. Along with the obvious effects of sleep deprivation, such as fatigue and difficulty maintaining attention, inadequate sleep contributes to irritability and depression. Studies of children and adolescents have found that sleep deprivation can increase impulsive behavior and can be a factor in delinquency. One interpretation of all these findings is that in teens, the parts of the brain involved in emotional responses are fully online, or even more active than in adults, while the parts of the brain involved in keeping emotional, impulsive responses in check are still reaching maturity. Such a changing balance might provide clues to a youthful appetite for novelty, and a tendency to act on impulse without regard for risk.

So why is it so often the case that, for many mental disorders, symptoms first emerge during adolescence and young adulthood? This question has been the central reason to study brain development from infancy to adulthood because mental illness is often seen as a developmental disorder having its roots in the processes involved in how the brain matures. It's not surprising that the behavior of adolescents would be a study in change, since the brain itself is changing in such striking ways. The fact that the teen brain is in transition doesn't mean it's somehow not up to par. It's simply different from both a child's and an adult's in ways that may equip youth to make the transition from dependence to independence.

The capacity for learning at this age, an expanding social life, and a taste for exploration and limit-testing may all, to some extent, be reflections of age-related biology. Understanding the changes taking place in the brain at this age presents an opportunity to intervene early in mental illnesses that have their onset at this age. Research findings on the brain may also serve to help adults understand the importance of creating an environment in which teens can explore and experiment while helping them avoid behaviors that are destructive to themselves and others. The mind-body connection is perhaps at its most sensitive during the adolescent years, and how we interact with and respond to teens' behaviors may shape that connection for the rest of their lives.

Attention Deficit Hyperactivity Disorder

Attention deficit hyperactivity disorder (ADHD) is one of the most common childhood brain disorders and can continue through adolescence and adulthood. Brain imaging studies in children with ADHD have revealed that the brain matures in a normal pattern but is delayed, on average, by about three years. The delay is most pronounced in brain regions involved in thinking, paying attention, and planning. Symptoms include difficulty staying focused and paying attention, difficulty controlling behavior, and hyperactivity (over-activity). These symptoms can make it difficult for a child with ADHD to succeed in school, get along with other children or adults, or finish tasks at home.

Inattention, hyperactivity, and impulsivity are the three key behaviors of ADHD. It's normal for all children to be inattentive, hyperactive, or impulsive sometimes, but for children with ADHD, these behaviors are more severe and occur more often. To be diagnosed with the disorder, a child must have symptoms for six or more months and to a degree that is greater than other children of the same age. According to the Institutes of Mental Health, the following are the key behaviors and symptoms of ADHD.

Children who have symptoms of inattention may

- Be easily distracted, miss details, forget things, and frequently switch from one activity to another.

- Have difficulty focusing on one thing.

- Become bored with a task after only a few minutes, unless they are doing something enjoyable.

- Have difficulty focusing attention on organizing and completing a task or learning something new.

- Have trouble completing or turning in homework assignments, often losing things (e.g., pencils, books, notes) needed to complete tasks or activities.

- Not seem to listen when spoken to.

- Daydream, become easily confused, and move slowly.

- Have difficulty processing information as quickly and accurately as others.

- Struggle to follow instructions.

Children who have symptoms of hyperactivity may

- Fidget and squirm in their seats.

- Talk nonstop.

- Dash around, touching or playing with anything and everything in sight.

- Have trouble sitting still during dinner, school, and story time.

- Be constantly in motion.

- Have difficulty doing quiet tasks or activities.

Children who have symptoms of impulsivity may

- Be very impatient.

- Blurt out inappropriate comments, show their emotions without restraint, and act without regard for consequences.

- Have difficulty waiting for things they want or waiting their turns in games.

- Often interrupt conversations or others' activities.

Children mature at different rates and have different personalities, temperaments, and energy levels. Most children get distracted, act impulsively, and struggle to concentrate at one time or another. Sometimes, these normal factors may be mistaken for ADHD. ADHD symptoms usually appear early in life, often between the ages of three and six and, because symptoms vary from person to person, the disorder can be hard to diagnose. Parents may first notice that their child loses interest in things sooner than other children, or seems constantly "unfocused" or "out of control." Often, teachers notice the symptoms first, when a child has trouble following rules, or frequently "spaces out" in the classroom or on the playground.

No single test can diagnose a child as having ADHD. Instead, a licensed health professional needs to gather information about the child, and his or her behavior and environment. A family may want to first talk with the child's pediatrician. Some pediatricians can assess the child themselves, but many will refer the family to a mental health specialist with experience in childhood brain disorders such as ADHD. The pediatrician or mental health specialist will first try to rule out other possibilities for the symptoms. For example, certain situations, events, or health conditions may cause temporary behaviors in a child that seem like ADHD. Currently, available treatments aim at reducing the symptoms of ADHD and improving functioning. Treatments include medication, various types of psychotherapy, education and training, or a combination of treatments.

Child and Adolescent Depression

To a great extent, good mental health depends on how we perceive events and how we handle the stress in our lives. This may be even more critical in children and adolescents because they don't have the necessary life experiences and have not yet learned to cope with stress effectively. Even small problems can become so painful that they lead to failure in school, drug abuse, violent behavior, or suicide.

Sadly, as many as two-thirds of all young people who need help for mental health disorders never get it. This is unfortunate because prompt attention and treatment can reduce both the duration and severity of mental health disorders and keep them from recurring. The cost to society is great since untreated mental health disorders during earlier years can easily manifest themselves as chronic emotional disorders throughout adult life.

In the past two decades, depression in children has been taken more seriously. Depressed children often pretend to be sick, refuse to go to school, cling to a parent, or worry that the parent may die. Older children tend to sulk, get into trouble at school, become negative, and feel misunderstood. Because normal behaviors vary from one childhood stage to another, it can be difficult to tell whether a child is just going through a temporary phase or is suffering from depression. If a visit to the pediatrician rules out physical illness, the doctor will probably suggest that the child be evaluated by a psychiatrist who specializes in the treatment of children.

Among both children and adolescents, depression is often misdiagnosed as normal mood swings associated with development, common anxiety, or social problems. Not recognizing and treating depression early can have far-reaching effects that lead to physical illness, substance abuse, and suicidal behavior. If a child or adolescent experiences five or more of the following symptoms within the same two week period, it could indicate major depression.

- Frequent episodes of sadness or empty feelings.
- Irritability, especially over insignificant things.
- Marked loss of interest in almost all activities.
- Insomnia or sleeping too much.
- Feelings of worthlessness, guilt, or hopelessness.
- Difficulty thinking, concentrating, or making decisions.
- Sudden loss of interest in school.
- Significant changes in weight.
- Unexplained crying or outbursts.
- Loss of interest in friends.
- Alcohol or substance abuse.
- Thoughts of death, especially suicide.
- Increased bouts of anger or hostility.
- Greater than normal fatigue and loss of energy.
- Reckless behavior.
- Relationship problems.

During their early years, boys and girls are equally at risk for depression. Once children reach puberty, however, girls are twice as likely as boys to develop depressive disorders, especially when there's a family history of depression or if one of the parents experienced depression at an early age. According to the National Institute of Mental Health, the greatest risk factors for depression in young people include: loss of a parent or loved one, breakup of a romantic relationship, attention or learning disorders, chronic illness, physical or mental abuse, sexual abuse, and trauma such as a natural disaster.

Child and Adolescent Bipolar Disorder

Although it is less common in children than in adults, bipolar disorder can also affect very young children and adolescents. As with depression, symptoms may be mistaken for normal emotions and behaviors that are typical of that age group. But unlike normal and temporary mood swings, bipolar disorder significantly impairs a child's ability to function in school, at home with the family, or with friends. Statistics show that 20 to 40 percent of adolescents with major depression develop bipolar disorder within five years after the onset of their depression.

According to the National Institute of Mental Health, bipolar disorder is a serious mental illness characterized by recurrent episodes of depression, mania, and other mixed symptom states. These episodes cause unusual and extreme shifts in mood, energy, and behavior that interfere significantly with normal, healthy functioning.

Manic symptoms include:

- Severe changes in mood, either extremely irritable or overly elated.
- Overly inflated self-esteem; grandiosity.
- Increased energy.

- Decreased need for sleep, ability to go with very little sleep, or no sleep for days without tiring.

- Increased talking, talking too much, or talking too fast; changing topics too quickly; cannot be interrupted.

- Distractibility; attention moves constantly from one thing to the next.

- Increased goal-directed activity or physical agitation.

- Disregard of risk; excessive involvement in risky behaviors or activities.

Depressive symptoms include:

- Persistent sad or irritable mood.

- Loss of interest in activities once enjoyed.

- Significant change in appetite or body weight.

- Difficulty sleeping or oversleeping.

- Physical agitation or slowing down.

- Loss of energy.

- Feelings of worthlessness or inappropriate guilt.

- Difficulty concentrating.

- Recurrent thought of death or suicide.

Symptoms of bipolar disorder in children and adolescents manifest themselves through a variety of different behaviors. Unlike adults, children and adolescents tend to be more irritable and prone to destructive outbursts than to euphoria. When they become depressed, they may have more physical complaints such as headaches, muscle aches, stomach pains, or tiredness, frequent absences from school or poor performance on tests, talk of or efforts to run away from home, irritability, complaining, unexplained crying, social isolation, poor communication, and extreme sensitivity to rejection or failure.

Other symptoms may include alcohol or substance abuse and difficulty with relationships.

According to the National Institute of Mental Health, existing evidence shows that bipolar disorder beginning in childhood or early adolescence may be a different, possibly more severe form of the illness than it is in older adolescents and adult-onset bipolar disorder. When the illness begins before or soon after puberty, it's often characterized by a continuous, rapid-cycle, mixed symptom state that may co-exist with conduct disorder (CD) or disruptive behavior disorders like attention deficit hyperactivity disorder (ADHD). In contrast, adolescent bipolar disorder tends to occur suddenly and have a more episodic pattern with relatively stable periods.

Researchers are now warning that a child or adolescent who appears depressed and/or exhibits severe ADHD-like symptoms, with excessive temper outbursts and mood changes, should be evaluated immediately. This is especially critical if there's a family history of bipolar disorder. Evaluation by someone with experience in bipolar disorder is important because medications for ADHD may actually worsen manic symptoms.

Once the diagnosis of bipolar disorder is made, the treatment of children and adolescents is based mainly on experience with adults and involves mood stabilizers, most typically lithium and/or valproate, which is often effective in controlling mania and preventing recurrences of manic and depressive episodes. Other treatments include various forms of psychotherapy to complement medical treatment.

Post-Traumatic Stress Disorder (PTSD)

Following a traumatic experience such as a natural disaster, physical or sexual abuse, or serious illness or injury, a child or teen may suffer severe emotional distress. While it's normal to react by withdrawing or feeling depressed or jumpy, reactions that last more than a month and are strong enough to affect day-to-day functioning are diagnosed as Post Traumatic Stress

Disorder or PTSD. Three factors have been shown to raise the chances that children will get PTSD. These factors are: how severe the trauma is, how the parents react to the trauma, and how close or far away the child is from the trauma. Children and teens who go through the most severe traumas tend to have the highest levels of PTSD symptoms. The PTSD symptoms may be less severe if the child has more family support and if the parents are less upset by the trauma. Lastly, children and teens who are farther away from the event report less distress.

Other factors can also affect PTSD. Events that involve people hurting other people, such as rape and assault, are more likely to result in PTSD than other types of traumas. Also, the more traumas a child goes through, the higher the risk of getting PTSD. Girls are more likely than boys to get PTSD. Another question is whether a child's age at the time of the trauma has an effect on PTSD. Researchers think it may not be that the effects of trauma differ according to the child's age. Rather, it may be that PTSD looks different in children of different ages.

According to the US Department of Health and Human Services (DHHS), about 30 percent of children who experience a traumatic event develop PTSD. Most of these children will have severe symptoms in the first few days or weeks after the event. The majority resolves their reactions, but children who have never had previous traumatic experiences, who have very strong reactions, or whose support systems (parents and others) are very distressed by the event, are at higher risk. The DHHS lists some common reactions for different age groups and separates childhood PTSD into three main categories: re-experiencing trauma, avoidance, and hyper-arousal.

Age Five and Under	Age Six to Twelve	Age Thirteen to Seventeen
Fearful expressions	Isolation and withdrawal	Flashbacks
Clinging to parent		Substance abuse
Crying or screaming	Nightmares and/or insomnia	Antisocial behavior
Whimpering	Irritable or disruptive	Physical complaints
Moving aimlessly	Angry outbursts	Nightmares and/or insomnia
Thumb sucking	Not able to concentrate	Isolation or confusion
Bedwetting	Unfounded fears	Suicidal thoughts
Fear of the dark	Problems with schoolwork	Depression
	Depression	

1. **Re-experiencing trauma.** Upsetting thoughts, pictures, or feelings about the traumatic event just pop into the child's mind; he or she may relive the traumatic event through nightmares or through flashbacks when awake; reminders of the trauma may bring tears or other physical symptoms such as sweating, heart pounding, nervousness, or stomach upset.

2. **Avoiding reminders of the trauma.** Avoids or wants to avoid situations, activities, or locations that might be reminders; he or she may feel emotionally numb or detached—shutting down emotions to protect from painful feelings; may feel less close to friends and family; can feel hopeless about the future.

3. **Hyper-arousal.** Becomes jumpy or easily startled (overreacts to a sudden loud noise, for example); he or she may become hypersensitive to signs of danger; may seem irritable or angry more than usual; may have sleep problems and trouble concentrating.

As shown in the previous chart, depending on a child's age, he or she will react differently to a traumatic event. Reactions can be immediate or they may appear much later and may differ in severity. They cover a range of behaviors because people have unique personalities and different cultures have their own ways of reacting. Other reactions vary according to age. A common response is loss of trust; another is fear of the event reoccurring. Children with existing mental health problems or who have experienced other traumatic events may be more affected.

Some symptoms may require immediate attention. Contact a mental health professional at once if the child is experiencing flashbacks, racing heart and sweating, being emotionally numb, being very sad or depressed, or having thoughts of or attempting suicide. Adults are often the first line of defense in helping children deal with PTSD. Here are some things to do following any traumatic event.

- **Observe.** Be aware of changes in your child's behavior.

- **Talk.** Instead of avoiding conversation, speak openly about the traumatic event in a matter-of-fact manner. If this is too upsetting for you, seek support from others who are also coping.

- **Listen.** Ask your child about his or her feelings regarding the traumatic event and pay close attention to words, tone, and body language. Gently help to correct misunderstandings. Sometimes children feel guilt about what happened and mistakenly believe they are to blame. Younger children may have unrealistic ideas about how the trauma occurred.

- **Support.** Help your child focus on his or her strengths and talents, and to develop and use strategies for healthy coping with fears or anxiety.

- **Take care of yourself.** Parents and other caregivers need to have support for themselves and their own reactions and feelings after a child has experienced a traumatic event.

- **Ask for help.** If a child continues to have symptoms that interfere with normal activities, or if a child has behaviors that endanger himself or others, get professional help immediately.

Stress Management for Young Children

It's natural for children to worry, especially when scary or stressful events happen in their lives. Even the most well-balanced and happiest child will face a number of challenges and a few traumatic events that invariably cause stress, anxiety, and mild depression. Usually these resolve themselves and the child will quickly get back to normal. If stress symptoms persist, however, you need to identify the source and take appropriate action before things get more serious. And if that doesn't work, always consult a mental health professional to prescribe medication if needed or techniques designed specifically for children. The following strategies are effective in helping children and family members manage the stress in both their lives.

- **Establish a daily family routine.** Studies show that stress-free households and happy children have a family routine that includes eating meals together, a regular time for homework each afternoon or evening, and going to bed at a set time. Helping children wake up, go to sleep, and eat meals at regular times provides them a sense of stability.

- **Set boundaries and rules.** Children feel secure, reassured, and protected when parents establish firm guidelines. When you say no, do it with care and concern, or learn to say no in other ways such as "Yes, after your homework is done." Children also need to learn how to say no appropriately so that they will make good choices during their teenage years and later as adults.

- **Talk, listen, and encourage expression.** Listen to your children and encourage them to express feelings, especially if you sense that they may be overwhelmed or experiencing stress. Create opportunities to have your children talk, but don't force them. After a traumatic event, it's important for children to feel they can share their feelings and to know that their fears and worries are understandable. Keep these conversations going by asking them how they feel in a week, then in a month, and so on. Respect their feelings and reassure them that everyone experiences nervousness, fear, and anxiety.

- **Watch and listen.** Be alert for any change in behavior. Are children sleeping more or less? Are they withdrawing from friends and family? Are they behaving in any way out of the ordinary? Any changes in behavior, even small changes, may be signs that the child is having trouble coming to terms with the stressful event and may need support.

- **Reassure.** Stressful events can challenge a child's sense of physical and emotional safety and security. Take opportunities to reassure your child about his or her safety and well-being and discuss ways that you, the school, and the community are taking steps to keep them safe.

- **Connect with others.** Make an on-going effort to talk to other parents and your child's teachers about concerns and ways to help your child cope. You do not have to deal with problems alone; it is often helpful for parents, schools, and health professionals to work together to support and ensure the well-being of all children in stressful times.

Praise and Self-Esteem

Praise is important to raising a confident child. Self-esteem encompasses the way children feel about what they believe are their positive qualities, values, abilities, and worth as human beings. Helping them develop self-esteem will protect them from hurtful or wrong images and labels that other people express about them. It also insulates them from bullies, poor influences, and peer pressure to engage in risky behavior.

Some new research challenges the notion that praise is a good thing and suggests that too much praise is being passed around, causing some children to become bold, rude, and self-centered. But this research also agrees with earlier findings—that the context and content of praise are as important as the praise itself. Some parents praise just for the sake of praising. Others limit praise in an effort to raise responsible children. What researchers found most disappointing was that praise is not often used as a tool for motivating children as they enter and proceed through middle school and into high school.

Psychologists and educators agree that judicious use of praise helps children develop concepts of fairness, effort, competence, and achievement. For example, a parent might say, "I'm pleased that you got an early start on your science project." This simple statement includes the context or description of the situation that warranted praise (getting an early start) and the content of expressing appreciation ("I'm pleased.").

Using either descriptive or appreciative praise can help children develop self-confidence and self-motivation. It also makes them less likely to be dependent on the approval of someone who can be a bad influence. When children feel in control of their lives, they will make decisions based on what they themselves approve of.

Descriptive praise makes children feel good because it's free of evaluation and focuses on their accomplishments and your observations. It describes in detail what the child has done that warranted praise. For example, "That's great! You got all the toys back into the box without a single reminder," or "This is really good! Your picture has lots of bright colors that attracted my attention."

This type of praise focuses on specifics, is free of evaluation, affirms what's been done, and leaves room for the child to draw a conclusion about his or her accomplishment. "I feel proud for cleaning up my room," or "I am creative." The evaluation is internal and is appreciated by the child. The following are some suggestions on how to deliver praise that will help children feel good about themselves and reinforce behavior that you would want them to repeat in the future.

- **Be honest and mean what you say.** "I'm pleased with the way your effort has improved your math grade," rather than "This grade is terrific."

- **Offer praise along the way.** You can start praising your child's efforts long before the finish line. For example, "I see that your extra effort has helped you spell two more words correctly than you did in last week's test."

- **Build your vocabulary.** Try different words that help describe your child's accomplishments in a more concrete way such as, "That science project looks well-constructed," or "This paper makes me look at that subject in a new way."

- **Be specific.** Talk about your child's specific accomplishment in terms of his or her performance and real skills or talent. Say, "I like the way you organized and wrote your book report," not just "I'm proud of you."

Appreciative praise helps children understand how behavior affects others. It's also free of evaluation and gives you an opportunity to mention specific behavior and its positive effects. For example, you can say, "Thank you for helping with the grocery shopping. It made that errand easier." This type of praise expresses thanks for a specific behavior, describes the positive effect it had on your life or that of the family, tells what behaviors are helpful, and shares appreciation. Here are some things to keep in mind as you let your children know that their efforts are as important as their achievements:

- **Be sincere.** Children can tell when praise is genuine. "Thanks for being ready to leave on time for the movie. We're all looking forward to it."

- **Comment on what you saw.** Be specific and describe the action you observed. For example, "You really worked hard at helping your brother learn to tie his shoes. I won't have to worry that he'll trip over his laces."

- **Choose the right words.** Using lavish words like terrific, excellent, super, tremendous, fantastic, and awesome may sound good at first, but they are difficult to maintain. A child may then be pressured to always be terrific or excellent. Just as important, lavish praise may be a reminder of all the times that he or she was not rewarded with appreciation, or may bring to mind the times when he or she wasn't so terrific or excellent at all. The compliment then becomes false praise.

When it comes to praise, being balanced is the best approach. Treat praising in the same way you would like to hear yourself being praised. At work, if you live on a steady diet of, "You're terrific!" "What a genius!" or "Great job!" you would have no way of knowing how you can improve or what you should keep doing that pleases your boss. Whereas, "That's a nice layout; the colors really pop," makes you feel good about a job well done and describes an accomplishment you can build on.

Likewise, sincere praise about children's accomplishments will help them become the confident, competent, and responsible adults you want them to be.

Coping with School

There aren't many milestones in a child's life more significant than beginning school. For some children it's also a traumatic and stressful time because he or she is suddenly exposed to a new and sometimes frightening environment. It's often the first major separation from the secure and familiar world of home and family. How you handle this turning point is important to your child's future attitude about school and the self-confidence he or she will need throughout life.

Preparation—yours and your child's—can make that first milestone less stressful. To help children cope with those first few days of school, the following suggestions can ease the transition and make school an exciting part of life.

- **Talk about school in a positive way.** Answer any questions your child may have about what to expect in school, how he or she will get there, what to do on the school bus, what they'll do after school, etc. Children are understandably nervous about this new experience, so it's up to parents to reassure them and convince them that it will be something positive and exciting. The more enthusiastic you are, the more your child will look forward to it.

- **Make the first day special and exciting.** For a young child, this is probably the first time that he or she will feel separated from home and family. That itself may be traumatic. To ease the fear, parents should make the first day special by talking up how great school will be and how they look forward to hearing all about this wonderful experience when the child comes home.

- **Allow more free time at home.** Until now, your child had all day to play. To avoid having your child associate school with a loss of free time, make sure that he or she has enough play time at home and on weekends.

- **Praise your child's schoolwork.** Always be positive and give praise when your children bring home schoolwork. Tell them that they're doing great in school in order to reinforce good behavior and good performance.

- **Keep it normal.** Once the novelty of school becomes routine, treat it as something that's expected as part of life. If your child appears nervous about something going on at school, discuss his or her concern and resolve the issue immediately before it affects your child's attitude and behavior.

- **Avoid comparisons.** It seems some parents can't help but make comparisons between children. However, few things are worse for a child's self-image than to hear that his or her sibling is doing much better in school, sports, or life in general. Each child is different, and each child needs to progress in his or her our own way.

If after a few days none of these suggestions work, and the child still seems distressed or fearful about school, there may be a deeper problem. In that case, it's best to get counseling from a school psychologist or a mental health expert who can offer expert advice. In most cases, however, children will make a natural transition and begin to feel more comfortable away from home, especially as they make new friends. Before you know it, children will overcome their initial anxiety and make school a normal and enjoyable part of their lives.

Coping with Grief and Death

For young children, the death of a parent has to be one of the most traumatic events in their lives because their main source of support is gone. They may even feel responsible, angry, or guilty. As they get older, if their loss stays with them, they are statistically more likely to experience a greater incidence of depression, anxiety, and substance abuse than children who grow up with two living parents. And even though they begin to understand that what lives must also die, it doesn't make it any easier.

School-aged children are interested in the physical aspects of death and dying. By the age of nine, nearly all children realize that death is inevitable and irreversible, but they don't think it will happen to them any time soon. Adolescents have a more mature concept of death, but like younger children don't believe it will happen to them. The "I am invincible" attitude is one of the factors that leads to risk-taking behavior.

A child's age and developmental level influences the way he or she understands death and expresses grief. Between birth and the teenage years, children develop an understanding of the concept of death and many related beliefs. According to Federal Occupational Health (FOH), a service unit within the Department of Health and Human Services, the following are typical responses to loss depending on a child's age and stage of development, from birth to age seventeen.

Infants and toddlers (birth to two years)

While an infant will not understand the death of a loved one, his or her behavior may be affected by changes in routine or the grief of others around him or her. Common reactions may include fussiness, clinginess, disrupted sleep patterns, and physical reactions such as biting, hitting, or pushing to express frustration and confusion. Around the age of two, a child may start to show a slight comprehension of the loss, but his or her reaction will tend to be egocentric—in relation to self.

Preschoolers (three to five years)

Preschoolers typically have a poor sense of time and

permanence and may view the death as reversible. He or she may think death is the same as going to sleep and the child may suddenly fear nighttime, getting ready for bed, or falling asleep. A child may also experience confusion, bad dreams, and general agitation. Regression in the form of thumb sucking, bedwetting, and tantrums may also occur. Misunderstandings about what death is may be common; a child may ask repeated questions with little understanding of the answers. Sometimes a child at this age will worry intensely that someone else close to him or her will die soon.

School-aged children (six to twelve years)

Younger school-aged children tend to understand death in a more concrete way. This is around the age where a child will come to understand that death is final. He or she may become very interested in the process of death, wondering, for example, what happens to the body after death or asking repeated questions about the deceased. Children are now capable of suffering from sorrow, anger, and denial, but they still may not view death as something that can happen to them. Younger school-aged children may attempt to avoid emotional pain at all costs; they may play, act silly, or become easily distracted whenever the deceased is spoken of.

Older school-aged children are generally mature enough to know something is wrong when a death occurs. They understand that death is final and irreversible, and it can happen to anyone—including them. The child may reach out to you or other adults for help in dealing with intense feelings, or he or she may become withdrawn, quiet, or irritable—often a sign that he or she is fearful of loss or change. Children may also become self-conscious about expressing their feelings, or they may cover up the grief by joking about the experience. This may signal that they are confused about what to say or how to act.

Teenagers (thirteen to seventeen years)

Teens understand death much as adults do, but they have fewer coping skills. Because teens are already struggling to find their own voice and identity, the death of a friend or loved one may leave them feeling more bewildered and confused. They may not be emotionally ready to deal with the death alone, yet they may struggle or refuse to share feelings or ask advice from parents or other adults.

Reactions to death can vary from sadness, regression, and despair to severe depression or uncontrolled behavioral problems such as angry outburst and rebellion. Sometimes feelings of sadness are interrupted by periods of playing and laughing, so parents should not be overly concerned about seemingly inappropriate behavior. To help a child overcome an event that can severely disrupt mind-body reactions, here are a few strategies to help ease the pain and sadness.

- **Encourage children to ask questions.** Children are inquisitive by nature. They want to ask questions and they need to have answers. In many ways, their fantasies about death and dying could be much worse than the reality of death itself. Don't be afraid to answer questions that will help your child understand what happened. Talk on their level, but be honest. For example, telling a child that someone who died has gone to sleep will make them afraid of going to bed at night. If the child is afraid, talking will help lessen fears and anxieties and make him or her feel like part of the family.

- **Avoid other life changes.** Death is a traumatic life experience for anyone, but especially for a child. So the most important thing that you can do for at least a few months is to make your child feel safe, secure, and stable. And that means no unnecessary moving, no family disruptions, no changing schools, no sudden lifestyle shifts, and no other major life changes that could make your child feel insecure. Family disruptions can intensify the stress reactions that trigger physical and emotional disorders, so try to avoid them until your child seems back to normal.

• **Express your feelings freely.** Regardless of how much you want to protect your child from pain, he or she needs to feel included in the grieving process. Inclusion makes your child feel like a part of the family and gives him or her a sense of belonging in every sense of the word. Naturally, you don't want to be so emotional that you frighten your child into panic; but at the same time you don't want to exclude your child from what should be an intimately shared experience.

As parents, we all want to shield our children from the pain of death and dying. But trying to protect them from what's natural and inevitable is detrimental to their understanding of life. The grief a child experiences is often deep and similar to that in adults and may last several months. Therefore, good communication is essential to helping children cope with loss. As time goes by, eating, sleeping, and behavior patterns return to normal, and their experience will make them better able to deal with loss the next time.

Talking About War and Terrorism

Before talking to children about war, parents should take time to think about the issue themselves and consider what it means to their family. Each family is unique, with its own special history and past experiences about loss, trauma, and war. Let children know in language they can understand that the decision to go to war was a difficult and serious one that took a lot of time to decide. Explain that war is intended to keep them safe and to prevent bad things from happening in the future.

Because what we know about war changes every day, children may have questions on more than one occasion. Issues may need to be discussed more than once. New events may need to be clarified for children. Parents should remain flexible and be open to new questions. In some countries, the threat of war and terror is part of life, so parents need to help children cope with the stress and anxiety of not being sure whether they will be safe from one day to the next. Here are some ways to address the concerns and needs of children.

- **Be open, available, and positive.** Create an environment that supports communication that includes conversations about war and terrorism. Use family times such as mealtimes to talk about what's happening in the world. Follow the conversation with a favorable story or a pleasant family activity to help return the children to established routines.

- **Don't overexpose your children.** Serve as a protective shield against the images of war, particularly those on television. Children should not be overexposed to the sights and sounds of war. Even if you're in the room, children should be shielded from images of war, however brief they may be. If children want to talk about things they've seen and heard related to war or terrorism, discuss their thoughts and feelings.

- **Reassure children they are safe.** Make it a point to tell children that war will not be dangerous to their home or to their neighborhood. Explain what things are being done in their community, the state, and nationally to promote safety. Separate fact from fiction by answering their questions honestly. Listen to their concerns and address them in a calm and reassuring manner.

- **Stick to everyday routines.** Don't change family rules or disrupt normal schedule for meals, bedtime, play, etc. Sudden changes will make them feel that something's wrong and cause stress and anxiety. The more you stick to routines, the less stress your child will feel.

- **Spend extra time with your children.** Stay connected with your children by getting more involved. It doesn't matter whether it's playing games outside, reading together indoors, or just cuddling. A little extra support goes a long way to helping them feel safe and secure. Be sure to tell children they are loved.

Dealing with Anger

There are four basic childhood emotions: joy, sadness, fear, and anger. Increasingly, stresses dealing with abuse, divorce, the economy, and social issues are creating an environment in which children feel alienated, frustrated, and angry. When anger becomes intense, it can lead to rage, which often manifests itself as withdrawal or violent behavior.

Recognizing anger is the first step in dealing with it. Changes in your child's thoughts and feelings will lead to changes in their body language and their behavior. These could include: clenched fists, tightness or tenseness in their body, verbal outbursts, a particular facial expression, or physical violence. When anger takes over, it can come in different forms, from a verbal outburst to being physically aggressive and causing damage to furniture. Anger can sometimes make children act in a way that's harmful to themselves or others. For example, punching walls or hitting someone. Try to make the surrounding environment as safe as possible if this happens.

One of the dangers of chronic childhood anger is that it can eventually lead to physical illness. A study published in the *Journal of the American Medical Association* found that young adults who scored high on tests designed to measure anger and hostility were already in the process of developing heart disease well before showing physical symptoms, and that those with the highest hostility scores had the greatest amount of plaque buildup in their coronary arteries. This was the first study to show a link between a physical disorder such as heart disease and emotions such as anger in young people.

What's obvious from the study is that the mind-body connection in young people is being severely compromised by emotions such as anger and, therefore, in order to prevent the child from developing diseases of adulthood, it's important to intervene as early as possible. The following are some suggestions.

- **Identify the early warning signs.** Work together with your child to try to find out what it is that's triggering the anger. Pay attention to how he or she is dealing with problems, because in many cases anger is simply an outward expression of failure, rejection, or frustration. Once you've isolated what's causing the anger, you'll be in a better position to curb it once it comes. Talk about strategies that you and your child can use against anger such as counting to ten or stopping to take a few deep breaths, and when you see the early warning signs, give your child a gentle reminder that anger may be trying to sneak up. This gives them the chance to try their strategies.

- **Don't judge children for their anger.** Help your children deal with anger by letting them know that the anger is the problem, not them. With younger children this can be fun and creative. Give anger a name and try drawing it. For example, anger can be a volcano that eventually explodes. How you respond to anger can influence how your child responds to anger. Making it something you do together can help you both.

- **Have specific goals.** Have an agreed goal to work toward, with a way of recognizing what you're achieving together. You could have a star chart on the wall and reward your child with stickers for keeping anger away for a whole hour, then gradually move to half a day, then a day, and so on.

- **Praise your child.** Positive feedback is important. Praise your child's efforts and your own efforts, no matter how small. This will build your child's confidence in the battle against anger. It will also help them feel that you're both learning together. The more time you spend on praising their efforts, the less time there is for punishment for failing.

- **Make good behavior a habit.** By reinforcing the child's good behavior with praise and rewards, you'll be conditioning your child's developing brain in a way that will alter bad behavior. Remember that habits are conditioned responses; and the more your child's brain is conditioned, the stronger those habits become.

- **Allow your child to freely express emotions.** Sometimes children lash out simply because of frustration that there's nowhere else to vent their feelings or concerns. By allowing your child to openly discuss, and even argue, without fear of reprisal is important if you want to keep the lines of communication open and the dialogue going.

Because a young brain is still forming, what seems trivial to adults can be significant for children. They simply can't deal with stress and with life issues in the same way. Anger is just a manifestation of that reality. The problem with uncontrolled anger is that it can lead to more serious emotional and physical problems and, according to experts, may be a symptom of other conditions, including ADHD, bipolar disorder, and depression. By working together to control bouts of anger and violence, the child will develop a sense of calmness when things go wrong, and learn that there are much better ways to deal with frustrations than just lashing out.

Stress Management with Preteens

As children approach their teenage years, they experience

confusing physical and emotional changes. This "in between" age—old enough to understand many adult subjects, yet young enough that brain development has not been completed—can be traumatic for both the preteen and parent.

Because this is an especially difficult period, parents should build a special rapport with their child so that communication is there when it's needed. Stress management is important during this time so that children can cope with the pressures of peer groups and alcohol and other drugs, as well as relationships with others. The city of Ruston, Louisiana health services developed some excellent guidelines for helping parents and preteens cope with stress and get through those tough years.

- **Rephrase comments to show you understand.** Sometimes called "reflective listening," this technique serves three important purposes: 1) it assures your child that you're hearing what he or she is saying; 2) it allows your child to "rehear" and consider his or her own feelings; and 3) it assures you that you correctly understand your child.

- **Be aware of face and body language.** Often, a child will assure you that he or she doesn't feel sad or dejected, but a quivering chin or glistening eyes will tell you otherwise. When words and body language are in conflict, always believe the body language.

- **Give nonverbal support and encouragement.** This includes a smile, hug, wink, pat on the shoulder, nodding your head, making eye contact, or reaching for your child's hand.

- **Use the right tone of voice.** Tone communicates as clearly as words. Make sure that the tone of your voice doesn't come across as sarcastic or all-knowing.

- **Use encouraging phrases to show your interest and to keep conversation going.** Phrases such as "Oh, really?," "Tell me about it," "It sounds as if you . . .," and "Then what happened?" are great for communicating to your preteen that you really care. If there's a pause in your conversation, use phrases such as these to encourage dialogue.

- **Give lots of (the right kind of) praise.** Look for achievement, even in small tasks, and praise your child often. You're more likely to get the behavior you want when you emphasize the positive, and your praise will help your child have positive feelings.

- **Praise effort, not just accomplishment.** Let your child know that he or she doesn't always have to win. Trying hard and giving one's best is a noble feat in itself.

- **Help set realistic goals.** If the child, or the parent, expects too much, the resulting failure can be a crushing blow. If a preteen who's an average or mediocre athlete announces that he plans to become the school quarterback, it might be wise to gently suggest that just making the team would be a wonderful goal and a success in itself.

- **Don't compare your child's efforts with others.** There will always be other children who are better or worse at something than your child, more or less intelligent, more or less artistic, etc. Your preteen may not know that a good effort will make you just as proud as a blue ribbon.

- **When correcting, criticize the action, not the child.** A thoughtless comment can be devastating to a child. A preteen still takes an adult's word as law, so parents should notice how they phrase corrections.

  Helpful example: "Climbing that fence was dangerous. You could have been hurt, so don't do it again."
  Hurtful example: "You shouldn't have climbed that fence. Don't you have any sense?

- **Make sure your child gets enough sleep.** A study of 5,000 adolescents, published in the *Journal of the American Academy of Pediatrics*, found that lack of sleep can lead to behavior that mimics psychological disorders. Sleep deprivation can often transform an otherwise normal child into a moody and sometimes withdrawn individual who gets stressed out much more easily over what should be insignificant events. Fatigue affects schoolwork, physical activities, and relationships, so make sure your child is getting all the sleep he or she needs. How much is enough? For toddlers, at least eleven hours plus two hours of naps per day; for preschoolers, eleven to twelve hours, with or without a nap; for preteens, ten hours; for teens, about nine hours.

- **Take responsibility for your own negative feelings.** One constructive way to share your own negative feelings about a situation is to use "I messages." I messages don't make children feel like they are under attack or that they are intrinsically bad.

  Helpful example: "Keeping the house neat is important to me. I get upset when you leave your books and clothes in the hall."
  Hurtful example: "You act like a pig sometimes. When will you learn to put things where they belong?"

- **Give your child real responsibility.** Children who have regular duties around the house know they're doing something important to help out. They learn to see themselves as a useful and important part of the team. Completing their duties also instills a sense of accomplishment.

- **Show your children you love them.** Hugs, kisses, and saying, "I love you" help your children feel good about themselves. Children are never too young or too old to be told that they're loved and highly valued. In families where parents are divorced, it's helpful if the nonresident parent also expresses love and support for the children. When the parent-child relationship is strong and loving, single parent families, including those where parents are widowed or unmarried can give their children the same basis for self-esteem as two-parent families.

Stress Management for Adolescents

The adolescent years are an especially tough period of life. Adolescents want to be liked, they're overly concerned about how they look, they're maturing sexually, their hormone levels are bouncing all over the physiological scale, and they're just beginning to think about what they want to do in life. One of the greatest times of stress for families is the onset of these vulnerable years.

For many families, these are years of turmoil and strife, a period of transition in which adolescents are honing their social skills while at the same time striving for independence and freedom. The frightening reality of drugs, AIDS, violence, and broken homes adds a real dimension to stress that makes being a teenager one of the greatest challenges a young person will face.

As parents we're equally affected, and we need to deal with both our teenager's stress as well as the stress we feel as a result of our teenager's stress. The first step in bringing some harmony back into our lives is to recognize that certain ideals and expectations we have for our children create stress. We may feel helpless as we watch them try to do things by themselves, often in ways that seem strange and controversial. This lack of control sets the stage for confrontation, intolerance, and tremendous distress. Here are some suggestions for parents to follow.

Suggestions for Parents

- **Give your undivided attention whenever your teenager wants to talk to you.** These moments may be rare, so take advantage of them. A good rule of thumb is to listen twice as much as you talk.

- **When you listen, listen calmly.** Keep the door open on any subject and permit free expression of ideas and feelings. Never overreact or make judgments, and don't preach. Always be fair, courteous, and respectful in your response.

- **Take an interest in your teenager's activities.** Respect his or her desire for individuality and independence. Keep the door open on any subject, even if you don't feel comfortable talking about it yourself.

- **Don't expect your teenager to follow rules and regulations the same way you do.** This is a time when young minds are forming rapidly and limits are tested. But adolescents need and want limits, as long as they're not too rigid.

- **Don't get upset when your teenager tells you he or she hates you.** It's a normal reaction to the limits you set for your child.

- **Don't blame yourself for your teenager's attitude.** There's no such thing as a perfect parent, and you'll only make things worse if you continue to blame yourself for conflicts.

- **Don't be judgmental.** This is the fastest way to have your child stop confiding in you. Even if you disapprove of your child's behavior, try to understand his or her feelings. Remembering what it was like when you were an adolescent helps you be more empathetic.

- **Help your adolescent learn stress and time management skills.** Organization and time management skills are often nonexistent during the teen years, and it's typical for young people to wait till the last minute to finish projects. One of the best ways to help is to teach them to break projects down into smaller parts and then work on those parts a piece at a time.

- **Continue to build your teenager's confidence and self-worth.** Encourage (but do not force) participation in sports, music, art, dance, or any other hobby or activity that may, to his or her surprise, be a natural gift. Your youngster's new interests will usually be an added source of conversation and sharing.

It's good to set limits and have rules, because all teenagers need those boundaries to learn respect and discipline and to feel a sense of security. However, parents who are too controlling or expect too much will create a family dynamic that is stressful and unhealthy for both parent and child. According to psychologists, giving your teenager some room to grow not only eases the emotional changes that accompany adolescence, it creates a home environment that encourages communication and respect. That in itself will create less stress for your teenager and, as a result, even less stress for you.

Signs and Symptoms of Suicidal Behavior

The Department of Health and Human Services has found that suicide is the third leading cause of death in ten-to-twenty-four-year-olds. Moreover, the National Institute of Mental Health found that among adolescents who develop major depressive disorders, as many as 7 percent may commit suicide in the young adult years. More troubling is the fact that many adolescent suicides may be disguised as accidents. It's impossible to know, for instance, how many fatal car accidents (the leading cause of adolescent death) are a means of committing suicide. The number of attempted suicides has also been linked to childhood stress. The following graph shows the lifetime history of suicide attempts versus the number of adverse childhood experiences (ACE). As the number of stressful life events increased from zero to seven or more, the history of suicide attempts rose dramatically from a low of 1.1 percent to a high of 35.2 percent (see Figure 11.1).

Figure 11.1: Adverse Childhood Experiences and Suicide Attempts

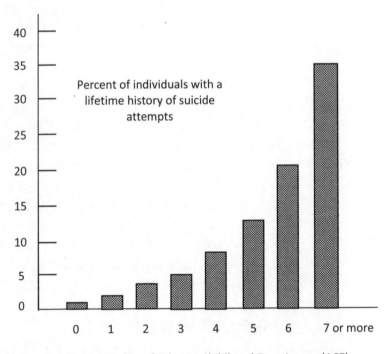

Percent of individuals with a lifetime history of suicide attempts

Number of Adverse Childhood Experiences (ACE)

Associations were found between ACE and many negative health behaviors, some of which may lead to suicidal behavior. For example, individuals with higher ACE scores were at greater risk of alcoholism, were more likely to marry an alcoholic, were more likely to initiate drug use and experience addiction, were more likely to have thirty or more sexual partners, engage in sexual intercourse earlier, and be more at risk of contracting AIDS, and were linked to a higher probability of both lifetime and recent depressive disorders.

In many cases, depression is the main trigger for suicide, and depression in young people is usually the result of repeatedly negative life events. The American College Health Association, for example, found that about 30 percent of college students reported feeling so depressed that it was difficult to function at some time in the past year. Students who were depressed were more likely to get poor grades, were more prone to smoke, were more likely to drink in order to get drunk, were more likely to engage in unsafe sex, and had a higher risk for suicide.

As adults, we view adolescence as a period of rebellion and transition, so we often don't recognize how serious the problem can be. For the adolescent, however, this period can be a very stressful time of concern about weight problems, acne, menstruation, late or early development, sexual arousal, school pressure, relationships, boredom, parental hassles, peer pressures, and money problems. By failing to recognize what are often cries for help, parents can actually intensify negative feelings and make the problem even worse.

Here are some warning signs to look for.

- Becoming withdrawn and isolated, especially from friends and family.

- Becoming less interested in personal appearance.

- Losing interest in school work, especially in grades.

- Losing or gaining too much weight.

- Becoming too self-critical, feeling like a failure, or feeling worthless.

- Becoming too preoccupied with death.

- Losing interest in activities that were once important.

- Becoming more accident prone.

- Becoming more apathetic and depressed.

• Having increased bouts of anger and hostility.

• Using alcohol or other drugs.

• Engaging in risky behaviors.

• Having feelings of hopelessness.

Thinking back to when you were a teenager, especially when sex hormones kicked in, you probably remember how even little things became blown-out-of-proportion crises. For parents and teachers, it's a challenge to steady the constant emotional highs and lows as teenagers bounce back and forth between feeling like children one minute and adults the next. To help get your teen through these troubled waters, parents need to be on a constant lookout for the emotional symptoms that usually precede suicidal thoughts.

Families need to keep the lines of communication open. If a young person knows that home is a place where feelings can be expressed freely and ideas shared and exchanged without criticism, that person will deal with stress and depression in a more positive way. As the results of a questionnaire given to adolescents showed, most chose "talking to a friend" as the single most important act they could do to lessen the threat of suicide. Communication is the key. If we put stress into words, we begin to interact with one another and develop a bond that has a tremendous effect on our ability to cope.

When teenagers were asked what their biggest sources of anger and frustration were, most responded "not being understood" and "not being listened to." Parents often find it impossible to listen to and communicate with teenagers because of personality clashes and the generational differences between them. But although the teenage years are a trying time for both parents and teenagers, it's also the most critical time of life to keep tuned in to each other.

Because the young brain is malleable, and neural connections are still growing, the way we interact with our children can determine how healthy they are, both physically and mentally, for the rest of their lives. We need to be aware of stages of child development so that we don't expect too much or too little from them. We should help our children set realistic goals based on their talents and limitations and then help them achieve their potential. We must love them unconditionally and teach them to love as well as respect others. And we should discipline fairly and consistently, but always allow them to express their thoughts and feelings so that they remain open to communication. Caring for a young mind early on will guarantee a healthy body and a powerful mind-body connection throughout life.

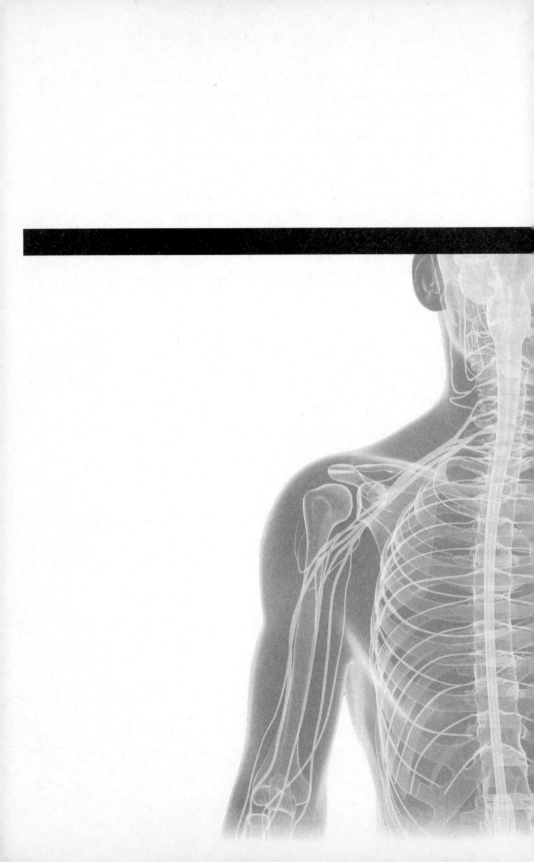

APPENDIX A

Time Management and Stress

Poor time management is one of the biggest factors in causing stress, particularly job stress and burnout. Lack of time management skills creates stress because we find ourselves in a constant battle to finish what needs to be done and enjoy the things we really want to do. When we feel like we're spinning our wheels and accomplishing little, we find ourselves stressed out and frustrated because every aspect of our lives seems to be dictated by the constraints of time.

Learning time management skills can make the difference between our hating work and enjoying it because these skills help us organize our life in a way that allows us to organize our day-to-day tasks in a way that makes us more efficient and productive. And when we become more productive, we're happier since we have more time for ourselves and our family. We also feel better about ourselves because we don't experience the physical effects of chronic stress so common in people with poor organizational skills.

Time Management Skills Test

The following time management skills test helps to identify trouble spots that prevent us from becoming successful time managers.

Read each statement and score it as follows: 1 = always; 2 = usually; 3 = sometimes; 4 = rarely. A scoring key at the end of the test will indicate how good a time manager you really are.

Statement	1	2	3	4
I meet assignment deadlines.	☐	☐	☐	☐
I keep a daily "to-do" list.	☐	☐	☐	☐
I make time to get away from the office.	☐	☐	☐	☐
I write down specific goals and objectives.	☐	☐	☐	☐
I set aside time each day for planning.	☐	☐	☐	☐
I create schedules and try to keep them.	☐	☐	☐	☐
I feel that I have control over my activities.	☐	☐	☐	☐
I have a clear idea of what my day will be like.	☐	☐	☐	☐
I am able to clear my desk by the end of the day.	☐	☐	☐	☐
I set priorities for all my tasks.	☐	☐	☐	☐
I include others in decision-making.	☐	☐	☐	☐
I have no problem delegating responsibilities.	☐	☐	☐	☐
I begin working on projects early.	☐	☐	☐	☐
I am able to reschedule low priority tasks.	☐	☐	☐	☐
I feel that I am efficient and well-organized.	☐	☐	☐	☐
I am clear about my duties and responsibilities.	☐	☐	☐	☐
I know how much time I spend on various tasks.	☐	☐	☐	☐
I leave time available in case the unexpected happens.	☐	☐	☐	☐

Statement

	1	2	3	4
I schedule demanding tasks at my peak energy levels.	☐	☐	☐	☐
I finish one task before starting another.	☐	☐	☐	☐
I find ways to cut down on duplicated effort.	☐	☐	☐	☐
I keep up with new developments.	☐	☐	☐	☐
I am able to identify sources of stress.	☐	☐	☐	☐
I break large projects down into smaller projects.	☐	☐	☐	☐
I am able to say no when pressed for time.	☐	☐	☐	☐

Scoring key:

25–40: You are an excellent time manager.

41–55: You are a good time manager, but need to improve your skills.

56–100: You are a poor time manager and in danger of burning out.

If your test score tells you that you're a poor time manager, go back and identify the personality traits that are the sources of time-related stress. By focusing in on specific behaviors and attitudes that interfere with your ability to get organized, meet deadlines, and accomplish your job effectively, you will reverse time management problems quickly and easily. According to occupational psychologists, here are the most common areas that create time management issues:

- Not prioritizing tasks.
- Poor or sloppy scheduling.
- Not delegating.
- Taking on too much work.
- Not using a calendar to meet deadlines and organize work.

- Not reducing clutter and unnecessary paperwork.

- Having to be in total control.

- Procrastinating.

Time Wasters That Create Stress

If you spend some time thinking about all the things you do that waste time, you'd probably be surprised. A time waster is any activity or behavior that is not necessary and that prevents you from doing your job and accomplishing your goals. At the end of the workday, time wasters ruin performance, sap your energy, and create stress because they are one of the main contributors to poor time management.

You need to get into the habit of monitoring how much time you spend reading emails, talking on the phone, running errands, chatting with coworkers, etc. Once you identify the main culprits, you then need to determine if they're necessary and, if not, how they could be eliminated. The following are what experts agree are the worst time wasters.

- Telephone interruptions, especially nonbusiness calls.

- Taking on additional, but unnecessary, duties.

- Reading unnecessary emails and/or spam.

- Unorganized and/or untimed meetings.

- Inadequate or insufficient information.

- Cluttered and/or disorganized desk.

- Too many coffee or smoke breaks.

- Little or no delegation.

- Drop-in visitors.

- Surfing the web.

- Procrastination.

Time wasters are classified as either self-inflicted or external. Self-inflicted time wasters are the things you do yourself like not planning or prioritizing, not delegating, taking too many breaks, and procrastinating. Because these are things you do yourself, they are more easily controlled. External time wasters, like telephone calls, mail, and drop-in visitors, are more difficult to resolve because other people are trying to control your time.

With a little effort, and by using the suggestions at the end of this chapter, you can eliminate both types of time wasters. Eliminating even some of them will increase productivity to the point that you'll feel less stressed and finally have a sense of accomplishment. The more consistently you make changes in your daily behavior, the greater the conditioning process is and the easier it becomes to form good work habits.

Tips for Students

As a university professor, I see it every day: students who do poorly on exams, withdraw from classes, and sometimes drop out of school, simply because they never learned to manage their time. Many of them feel that there are not enough hours in the day or they're under too much pressure or there are too many distractions. When I question them about the use of their time, what I find is that in most cases they're overwhelmed by scheduling, planning, and organizing their activities and school work.

The following time management strategies are effective for anyone, but students in particular have unique issues and problems to deal with. Here are some specific suggestions that should help students manage their time better and, in the process, eliminate some of the stress in their lives. The final section in this chapter offers more general guidelines for time management.

Find your best study time. Because we all have unique biological clocks, we all function differently during various time of the day. Some of us are morning people, some night owls.

Our individual biological clocks dictate whether we're better off studying when we first get up in the morning or whether we're better off waiting until later in the evening. Although you can train yourself to study at any time of the day or night, you should find when your peak energy levels are so that you can make the most of that energy for maximum learning. To find your own peak energy levels, spend a few weeks testing out how you function at different times of the day and then study accordingly.

Establish a study space. Whether you live in a house or a one-bedroom apartment, you have to set aside your own study area. It could be a desk or a kitchen table, but it must be quiet and have good light. It's also important to always use the same area for studying because your brain will be conditioned to respond to a particular environment. That's why writers do their best writing when they have their own space. Ernest Hemingway would often do his writing while standing up, with his pad on top of a filing cabinet. That was his space and his brain responded to it. If you continually change where you study, your brain will never become conditioned to link your study area with study.

Make your study space conducive to study. To ensure successful learning, avoid distractions from noise, music, people, and activities. If you know that certain times will be especially noisy or active, eliminate them from your study schedule. Instead, schedule your study during periods of the day or evening you know will be most peaceful. Also, make sure that you have plenty of bright light because memory, concentration, and positive attitude are enhanced when you're exposed to light, especially natural daylight.

Use a time planner. Buy yourself a planner and include a list of your classes, exams, due dates, meetings, and social activities. Refer to it often to stay on track. Allow for unexpected interruptions, so leave a block of time available each day for unexpected meetings or sudden schedule changes. If an open block of time gets used, prioritize your other activities and reschedule tasks. By leaving yourself a little time each day, you'll become less anxious knowing that you'll always be able to schedule one more thing if you really need to.

Never study more than an hour at a time without a break. The average person begins to lose concentration after about an hour. A mistake many students make is cramming or studying too long at any one time. Instead of absorbing information, you'll actually be wasting a lot of time and effort because your brain is not capable of maintaining a high level of concentration without a break every so often. The rule should be to take a ten or fifteen minute break every hour or so. It's also a good idea to switch subjects between learning sessions because studies have found that studying the same subject for prolonged periods of time can decrease your concentration and your ability to learn. Study wisely.

Beyond those described above, there are several other specific time management rules for students to help them study much more effectively.

- **Tackle the most difficult assignments when you're the least tired.** In order to maintain concentration and learn new material, make sure you're well rested and energized. You'll eliminate a lot of duplicated and wasted effort. Never study while in bed, and never study if you're distracted by something else.

- **Exercise and eat well.** Staying physically fit does more than keep your body in shape; it keeps your mind sharp and helps you concentrate and focus. Good nutrition is also important in maintaining a healthy brain and a strong immune system.

- **Use flash cards.** I always urge my students to use flash cards for every class I teach. Flash cards are an effective way to boil vital material down into short and manageable bits of information. Carry them around with you and refer to them between classes, while waiting for someone, during breaks, etc.

- **Don't take too many classes.** I see this as a real problem, especially with freshman. A full-time load is twelve credit hours, and a normal load that most students take in order to keep on track for their major is fifteen credit hours. Some students will take eighteen or more credits, thinking that they can handle that kind of load, and then run into all kinds of issues. Unless you're a genius, or some of those courses are really easy, don't overwhelm yourself with too many classes.

Time Management Plan of Action

Everyone has his or her own individual weaknesses when it comes to managing time. So, in order to recognize and eliminate those weaknesses, write them down in a time management diary, which should include three categories:

1. The event or activity.
2. Its priority ranking (1 = important; 2 = less important; 3 = least important; 4 = not important at all).
3. The action you take.

By setting down on paper a time management plan of action, you'll see exactly where you need to concentrate your efforts. And by giving each task a priority ranking, you'll avoid the time problems associated with wasted effort that leads to job stress and burnout. It's impossible to practice time management without first knowing what it is that makes us so bad at accomplishing a certain amount of work in a given amount of time. Once we identify the problems and their sources, it's much easier to change our behavior and begin to work more efficiently.

This is where conditioning, habit formation, and the mind-body link come into play once again. By consciously practicing good time management activities, we'll break our old time management habits and condition ourselves to develop new and more effective behavior patterns. These will quickly become new habits.

Conditioning and habit formation are powerful forces in shaping behavior and attitudes. The skills we develop and the ways in which we organize our lives are made possible through positive reinforcement. Our brain responds to any kind of conditioning process in the same manner, whether it's perceptions or specific behaviors. The more effectively we manage our time, the less stress we feel and the more positive the conditioning process becomes. Eventually, good time management simply becomes a natural part of our lives.

At the end of each day, write down specific time wasters and distractions and make a list of strategies that will solve problems dealing with those time wasters. Here's an example of a simple time management plan of action.

Time Management Plan of Action   Date:

Activity	Rank	Action Taken
Get payroll information to office	1	Started
Set up next week's meeting with company XYZ	3	Delegated
Complete next month's work schedule	2	Started; delegated
Do employee evaluations	1	Started; completed
Rearrange office furniture	4	Postponed
Plan the company office party	2	Delegated

Notes:

Time Wasting Activity	Strategy to Eliminate
Reading all my emails	Delete anything that looks like spam or junk mail
Going through all my regular mail	Prioritize mail; discard junk mail and only read high priority mail
Long meetings that don't accomplish much	Set specific time limits; assign agenda items to individuals who will be responsible for them; be better prepared
Too many interruptions during the day	Screen calls; schedule daily activities better; delegate minor tasks

Effective Time Management Strategies

As I've described throughout this book, through conditioning and habit formation the mind can be molded into an instrument of self-healing. Time management is no different. The positive reinforcement of good time management triggers healthy physiologic responses because the better we manage our time, the less stress we feel.

Nothing comes easily at first, especially if we've spent years conditioning ourselves to think in a negative way. Our ingrained habits prevent us from seeing things in certain ways, and they certainly hold us hostage to the day-to-day routines that make change difficult. It's only through repetition that we shape our thoughts and behaviors in the manner we choose. Here are fifteen ways to develop good time management habits and achieve our number one goal of staying healthy and stress-free.

1. **Plan a week ahead.** At the beginning of each week, make a list of upcoming goals and objectives. This initial planning session, which gets the wheels rolling and makes further planning easier, shouldn't be a concrete schedule but a preliminary activity chart that can be referred to whenever needed.

2. **Prioritize.** After writing down activities, goals, and plans, give them a priority ranking as follows:

Priority #1: Top priority—activity or task needs to be done as soon as possible. Plan your schedule around the activity in order to meet deadlines.

Priority #2: High priority—not as urgent, but should be done soon. Important enough to be put high on the schedule.

Priority #3: Low priority—activity or task can wait until other higher priority activities are accomplished. Responsibility may be delegated to someone else if time is a factor.

Priority #4: Lowest priority—not important or necessary. Activity or task should be placed last on the list, eliminated, or given to someone else to do.

3. **Use a calendar or appointment book.** This is one of the best ways to help organize time and plan activities. Calendars and appointment books are organized in a way that makes scheduling easy, effective, and manageable.

4. **Know your biological clock.** The most efficient individuals are those who recognize when their high energy levels are and then adjust their schedules accordingly. In most cases, it's best to tackle the most demanding assignments first and leave the easier tasks for the end of the day. Scheduling work in this manner will make you feel good because you'll get the tough assignment out of the way and finish the day in a pleasant and refreshing way.

5. **Identify time wasters.** Activities like reading every piece of junk mail or talking to everyone who calls can take valuable time away from more important tasks

and leave you frazzled by the end of the day. Make a commitment to eliminate the least important activities or, if necessary, put them at the end of the list.

6. **Delegate.** In order to be a good time manager, you have to be a good delegator. One of the biggest sources of job stress comes from the belief that you have to do it all yourself. Being in total control is ineffective because it places the burden of doing everything on your shoulders. Take a good look at your daily and weekly schedule of activities and then decide which of those can be handled by someone else. If you're working longer hours than everyone else, chances are that you're taking on a disproportionate amount of responsibility yourself.

7. **Avoid multitasking.** Some of us can handle more than one task at a time; most of us can't. We're always starting things and then putting them aside to be finished later. Before we know it, we have such a pile of unfinished tasks that we begin to feel the pressure of mounting work. Bad priority assignments and procrastination are the biggest culprits. The rules to follow when faced with this dilemma are:

   • **Assign a priority rating to every task.** Reschedule, postpone, or eliminate low priority tasks. Begin high priority tasks immediately.

   • **Eliminate the tendency to procrastinate.** Don't delay something because it's unpleasant or time-consuming. If it needs to be done, start right away. Also, don't string lengthy assignments together. Intersperse long assignments with short ones to avoid boredom and fatigue.

8. **Take good notes.** Being able to solve problems, accomplish goals, or finish assignments often depends on information you receive on the spur of the moment.

Taking good notes helps keep information handy when needed. Good note taking is also helpful when jotting down things people tell you while you're away from your calendar or appointment book. So, always keep a pencil and small notepad in your pocket, handbook, or briefcase and get in the habit of using it.

9. **Learn to say no.** One of the best ways to get organized and avoid scheduling problems is to avoid saying yes to everything you're asked, especially if it's unnecessary. Not being able to say no when you need to is stressful because it makes you feel as if everyone but you is making the decisions.

10. **Leave some of your schedule open.** Always leave a block of time available on your calendar each day for emergency meetings, unexpected jobs, or sudden schedule changes. If an open block of time gets used for some reason, analyze your schedule again and free up another block of time by eliminating a lower priority activity or rescheduling it for another day. By leaving yourself with some available time each day, you'll become less anxious knowing that you'll always be able to schedule one more thing if you really need to.

11. **Keep deadlines.** Once you decide to do something, there are some things you can do to make sure deadlines are met. They are:

    • **Don't put off a project that has a specific deadline.** Procrastination just makes deadlines that much harder to meet.

    • **Don't ignore deadlines.** Write them down, know when they are, and be aware of how long you have until the deadline ends. As long as you have a handle on deadlines, you can work toward those deadlines in an effective way.

- **Break projects down into smaller parts and set individual deadlines for each part.** Taking things one step at a time helps you judge how well you're doing along the way. Meeting deadlines consistently will make you feel productive and give you the incentive and motivation to keep striving toward the final deadline. Breaking projects down really helps you stay on schedule because you'll be following a specific plan of action that keeps you on track.

- **Allow yourself a few minutes from work every two hours or so in order to catch your breath and clear your mind.** However, don't get in the habit of wasting time by taking breaks every thirty minutes to get a drink or stretch your legs. Set up a schedule of two hours work and ten minutes of break and then stick with it.

12. **Be decisive.** Effective decision-making doesn't necessarily mean waiting until you have every fact and piece of information possible before making that decision. There comes a time when you have to say to yourself, "I have the information I need and I can act now without having to waste any more time looking at anything else." The tendency is, the longer you wait and the more information you try to gather, the harder it is to make a final decision. To avoid this scenario, follow four steps:

- Write down the decision you have to make.

- List the most important facts or the most important information you need to make a good decision.

- Get those facts and that information as quickly as possible.

- Make a decision based only on those facts and that information.

13. **Improve reading and writing skills.** Basic to all effective time management is the ability to read quickly and write well. Effective reading begins with knowing what to read, what to skim, and what to ignore altogether. By eliminating any unnecessary reading material right away, you'll free up some of your time and give yourself a chance to fill your schedule with more important activities. Effective writing is necessary for time management because it allows you to spend less time thinking about how to write and more time thinking about what to write. Both reading and writing can be improved through self-study or by taking courses designed to enhance reading and writing skills.

14. **Use a reminder system.** No one, regardless of how good his or her memory is, can remember everything. In cases where you need to be reminded to follow up, use a system such as index cards or calendars that involves a daily check of all activities. Each day, check your index card file and make sure that your follow-up activities don't interfere with more important plans.

15. **Maintain control.** Being in control is as important in time management as it is in stress management. All the scheduling, planning, and organizing in the world isn't going to do any good unless you can keep control over distractions, disturbances, and other activities that disrupt your day. In order to stay on top of activities, do the following:

• **Avoid spending too much time on the telephone.** Chatting unnecessarily makes you lose touch of time and keeps you from staying on schedule.

• **Avoid unnecessary socializing.** While some socializing and taking breaks are essential for proper work attitudes, overdoing it wastes time and leads to bad habit formation. Spend ten to fifteen minutes

every few hours away from your work, but control
the tendency to lengthen breaks or take them
more frequently.

- **Avoid upward delegation.** In order to fully control
  your schedule, you need to prevent people from
  delegating work back to you. Poor time managers are
  not able to delegate work in a way that will keep it
  delegated until it's finished. Conversely, good time
  managers delegate responsibility in order to free
  up their schedules and won't allow subordinates to
  delegate it back to them.

- **Avoid getting directly involved in others' activities.**
  It's difficult to relinquish some responsibilities and
  duties, but in order to be in control you can't allow
  yourself to get involved with everything everyone
  is doing. After delegating, remove yourself from the
  situation and periodically check on progress. Being
  directly involved only takes time away from more
  urgent and important duties and creates feelings of
  resentment between worker and manager.

- **Avoid unorganized meetings and discussions.**
  Meetings should be well-planned and timed. Let
  people know exactly when the meeting will take
  place, how long it's going to last, what the meeting
  will be about, and what kinds of materials they need
  to read or prepare beforehand. It's important to have
  an agenda ready to go as soon as the meeting begins.
  If you and everyone involved are well-prepared ahead
  of time, meetings and discussions can be kept under
  control and to the point.

The *way* we do things often creates more time management
problems than *what* we do. When we get bogged down by
poor organization, procrastination, or inefficient use of time,
we create a toxic environment that leads to stress, burnout,

and eventually illness. By simply changing our attitudes and behaviors, we become much more efficient at whatever we do.

Each year, billions of dollars are lost because of financial mismanagement, decreased productivity, inefficiency, illness, absenteeism, and premature death due to job-related stress. More than ever, today's workers are at risk because the complexity of today's workplace has become so overwhelming. Dealing with stress by focusing on the reasons and the causes, then alleviating that stress through stress management strategies that concentrate on the link between mind and body is critical for health and productivity.

At any one time, a significant portion of the work force experiences physical and/or emotional health problems due to job stress. Sometimes the solution for both worker and manager is simply recognizing things that can be changed and those that cannot, and then working together to implement strategies for creating a stress-free work environment. The good news for workers who experience chronic stress is that just as the mind is often the source of health problems it is just as often the source of healing and continued good health. All we have to do is change the way we think and act on the job and our body will do the rest. The serenity prayer, credited to Reinhold Niebuhr from 1934, reflects that goal and contains within it a philosophy that enables us to relieve many of our job-related stress problems.

God, grant me

the serenity to accept the things I cannot change,

the courage to change the things I can,

and the wisdom to know the difference.

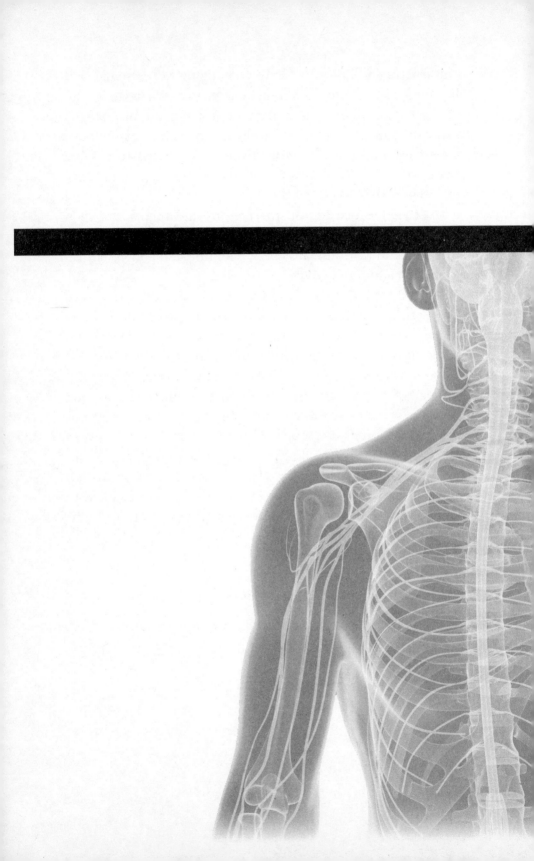

Health Assessment Quiz

How healthy do you think you are? Despite getting more information from more sources than ever, many of us don't know what to do to be as healthy as possible. Lifestyle is one of the most important factors affecting health, and it's estimated that 70 percent of all deaths could be reduced by simply changing lifestyle. The following test, designed by the Public Health Service of the US Department of Health and Human Services, is designed to tell you how much you are doing to stay healthy. Read each question and circle the number that corresponds to the following: 0 = almost never, 1 = sometimes, 2, 3, or 4 = almost always.

Cigarette Smoking

If you never smoke, enter a score of 10 for this section and go on to the next section on Alcohol and Drugs	10
I avoid smoking cigarettes.	2 1 0
I smoke only low tar and nicotine cigarettes or I smoke a pipe or cigar.	2 1 0

Smoking score: _____

Alcohol and Drugs

I avoid drinking alcoholic beverages, or I drink no more than one or two drinks a day.	4	1	0
I avoid using alcohol or other drugs, especially illegal drugs, as a way of handling stressful situations or the problems in my life.	2	1	0
I am careful not to drink alcohol when taking certain medicines (examples: medicine for sleeping, pain, colds, and allergies) or when pregnant.	2	1	0
I read and follow the label directions when using prescribed and over-the-counter drugs.	2	1	0

Alcohol and drugs score: _____

Eating Habits

I eat a variety of foods each day, such as fruits and vegetables, whole grain breads and cereals, lean meats, dairy products, dry peas and beans, and nuts and seeds.	4	1	0
I limit the amount of fat, saturated fat, and cholesterol I eat, including fat in meats, eggs, butter, cream, shortenings, and organ meats such as liver.	2	1	0
I limit the amount of salt I eat by cooking with only small amounts, not adding salt at the table, and avoiding salty snacks.	2	1	0
I avoid eating too much sugar, especially frequent snacks of sticky candy or soft drinks.	2	1	0

Eating habits score: _____

Exercise Fitness

I maintain a desired weight, avoiding overweight and underweight.	3	1	0
I do vigorous exercises for fifteen to thirty minutes at least three times a week (examples: running, swimming, and brisk walking).	3	1	0
I do exercises that enhance my muscle tone for fifteen to thirty minutes at least three times a week (examples: yoga and calisthenics).	2	1	2
I use part of my leisure time participating in individual, family, or team activities that increase my level of fitness (examples: gardening, bowling, golf, and baseball).	2	1	0

Exercise / fitness score: _____

Stress Control

I have a job or do other work that I enjoy.	2	1	0
I find it easy to relax and express my feelings freely.	2	1	0
I recognize early, and prepare for, events or situations likely to be stressful for me.	2	1	0
I have close friends, relatives, or other people I can talk to about personal matters and call on for help when needed.	2	1	0
I participate in group activities, such as community organizations, or hobbies that I enjoy.	2	1	0

Stress control score: _____

Safety

I wear a seat belt while riding in a car.	2	1	0
I avoid driving while under the influence of alcohol and other drugs.	2	1	0
I obey traffic rules and the speed limit while driving.	2	1	0
I am careful when using potentially harmful products or substances, such as chemicals, poisons, and electrical devices.	2	1	0
I make use of safety clothing and equipment at work and/or recreation (examples: gloves and lifejackets).	2	1	0

Safety score: _____

What Do Your Scores Mean?

Scores of 9 and 10: Excellent! Your answers show that you are aware of the importance of this area to your health. More importantly, you are putting your knowledge to work for you by practicing good health habits. As long as you continue to do so, this area should not pose a serious health risk. It is likely that you are setting an example for your family and friends to follow. Since you got a very high test score on this part of the test, you may want to consider other areas where your scores indicate room for improvement.

Scores of 6 to 8: Your health practices in this area are good, but there is room for improvement. Look again at the items you answered with Sometimes or Almost Never. What changes can you make to improve your score? Even a small change can often help you achieve better health.

Scores of 3 to 5: Your health risks are showing! Would you like more information about the risks you are facing and about why it is important for you to change these behaviors? Perhaps you need help in deciding how to successfully make the changes you desire. In either case, help is available.

Scores of 0 to 2: Obviously, you were concerned enough about your health to take the test, but your answers show that you may be taking serious and unnecessary risks with your health. Perhaps you are not aware of the risks and what to do about them. You can easily get the information and help you need to improve, if you wish. The next step is up to you.

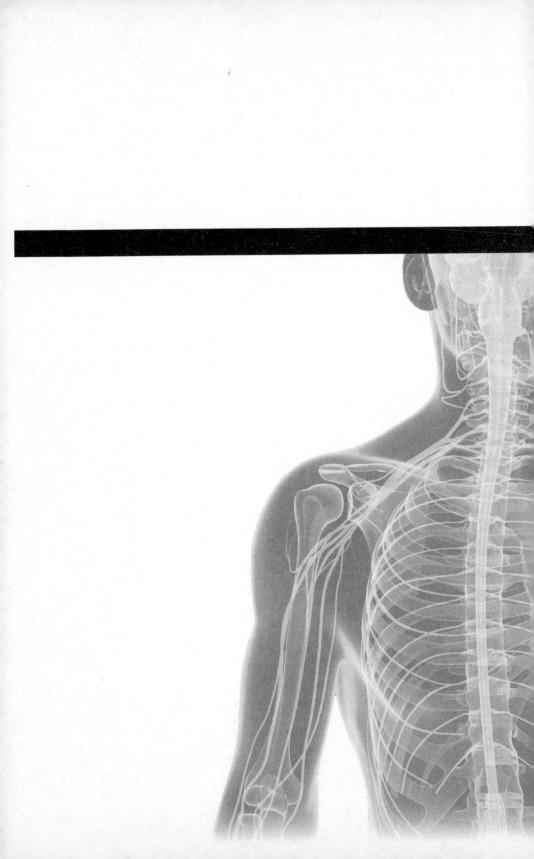

APPENDIX C

Family Stress Assessment Quiz

The National Institute of Safety and Health (NIOSH) has developed a family assessment questionnaire to determine if families are doing a good job of managing the stress in their lives.

Read the list of family statements below and ask yourself, "How well does this statement describe our family?" Rate each of the statements on a 1 to 5 scale (1 = your family is weak in that area and 5 = your family is extremely strong in that area). Following the quiz is some information about the scores.

Family Statement	1	2	3	4	5
Our family does many things together.	☐	☐	☐	☐	☐
Our family holds meetings whenever necessary.	☐	☐	☐	☐	☐
We encourage family members to help each other whenever possible.	☐	☐	☐	☐	☐
Our family is a priority.	☐	☐	☐	☐	☐
Our family allows members to participate in activities outside the family.	☐	☐	☐	☐	☐

Family Statement (continued)

	1	2	3	4	5
Our family members express appreciation for one another.	☐	☐	☐	☐	☐
Our family tries to look on the bright side no matter what happens.	☐	☐	☐	☐	☐
Our family is able to express a variety of feelings.	☐	☐	☐	☐	☐
Our family members are active in clubs and organizations.	☐	☐	☐	☐	☐
We can count on family and friends for help when we need to.	☐	☐	☐	☐	☐
Our family gets together with other families who have the same lifestyle.	☐	☐	☐	☐	☐
Our family is able to accept outside help when needed.	☐	☐	☐	☐	☐
We ignore criticisms of others about how we should function as a family.	☐	☐	☐	☐	☐
We believe there are more advantages than disadvantages to the way we live.	☐	☐	☐	☐	☐
Our roles in the family are shared.	☐	☐	☐	☐	☐
We believe that our lifestyle has made us better people and a stronger family.	☐	☐	☐	☐	☐
Our family doesn't let problems go unresolved.	☐	☐	☐	☐	☐
We relieve tension through sports, exercise, and relaxing.	☐	☐	☐	☐	☐
Our family tries to stay healthy by eating right, not smoking, and keeping active.	☐	☐	☐	☐	☐
Our family has many hobbies to help us manage stress.	☐	☐	☐	☐	☐

Characteristics of families who score high (3 to 5 per statement)

- **They do things as a family.** They work hard at keeping the family functioning. When under stress, it is very easy for family members to withdraw from each other. Just because families live under the same roof doesn't mean they do things together. Statements 1 to 4 are examples of families doing things together.

- **They build esteem in each other and themselves.** They show appreciation for each other and let other members know they understand. It's common for a family member's self-esteem to be affected when stress occurs. Families who do a good job of managing stress take care of themselves physically and mentally. Statements 5 to 8 are examples of families building self-esteem in each other.

- **They develop social support networks.** Families are better able to endure hardships if they reach out to the community instead of becoming isolated in it. Meeting new friends, joining clubs, and using community facilities are great ways to become involved. Statements 9 to 12 are examples of developing social support.

- **They enjoy the lifestyle they have chosen and cope better with hardships than those who are not satisfied with their way of life.** For example, a homemaker who enjoys that lifestyle and is supported by family and friends will feel less stress than a person who would rather be away from home but for various reasons cannot be. Statements 13 to 16 are examples of accepting one's lifestyle.

- **They develop and use a range of tension-reducing devices such as exercise, relaxation, and keeping involved in activities.** These techniques manage the tensions and conflicts that are part of family life. Statements 17 to 20 are example of reducing tension.

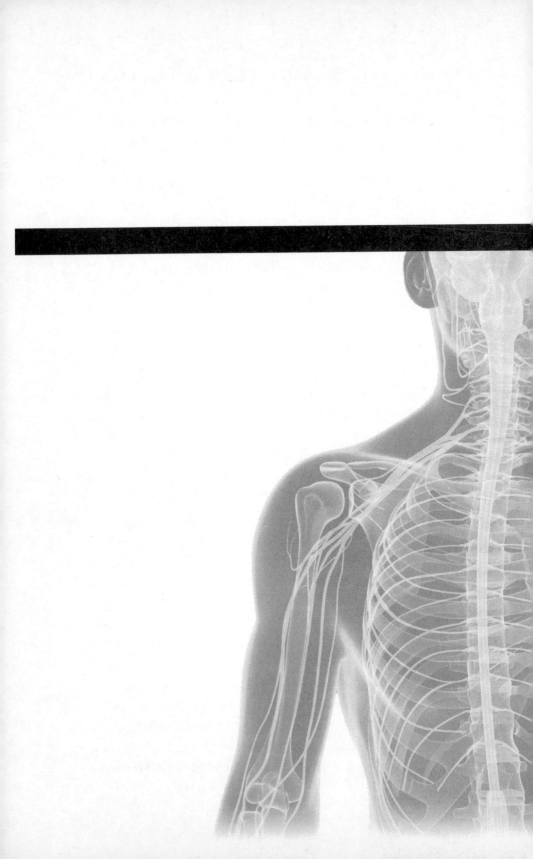

Health Screening Checklist

Take the following checklist to your doctor's office. Write down when you have any of the tests listed. Talk to your doctor about your results and write them down. Ask when you should next have the test. Write down the month and year. If you think of any questions, write them down and bring them to your next visit.

Test	Last test (m/y)	Results	Next test (m/y)	Questions for doctor
Weight/BMI				
Cholesterol				
HDL				
LDL				
Blood pressure				
Colon screening				
Blood sugar				
Thyroid				
STD's				
For women:				
Mammogram				
Pap smear				
Bone density				

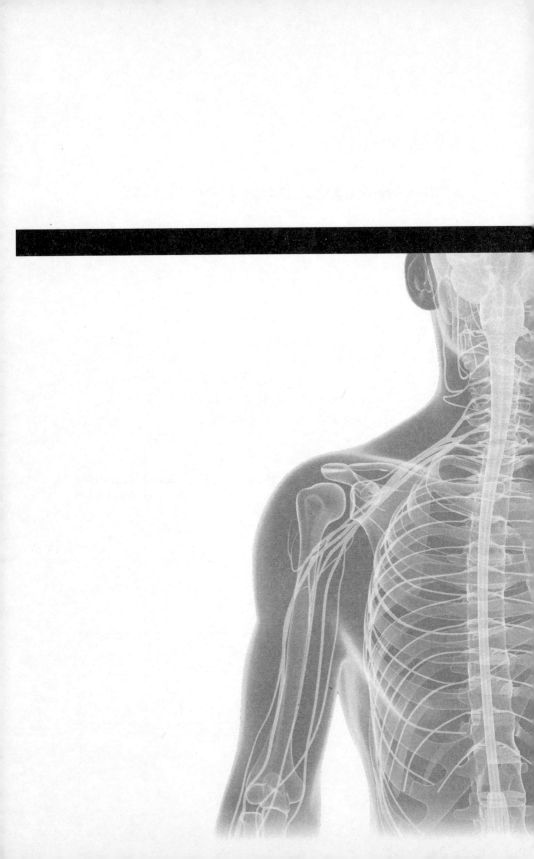

Endnotes

[1] Hollenstein, K., J. Kean, A. Bortolato, R. K. Cheng, A. S. Doré, A. Jazayeri, R. M. Cooke, M. Weir, and F. H. Marshall. 2013. Structure of class B GPCR corticotropin-releasing factor receptor 1. *Nature* 499:438-43.

[2] De Craen, A. J., P. J. Roos, A. de Vries, and J. Kleijnen. 1996. Effect of colour of drugs: Systematic review of perceived effect of drugs and of their effects. *BMJ* 313:1624-6.

[3] Pelletier, K. 1993. Between mind and body: stress, emotions and health in mind-body medicine. In *Mind Body Medicine: How to Use Your Mind for Better Health*, eds. D. Goleman and J. Gurin. New York: Consumer Reports Book.

[4] Epel, E. S., E. H. Blackburn, J. Lin, F. S. Dhabhar, N. E. Adler, J. D. Morrow, and R. M. Cawthon. 2004. Accelerated telomere shortening in response to life stress. *Proceedings of the National Academy of Sciences* 101(49):17312-5.

[5] Davis, A. 1999. Stress—It might be even worse than you think. *The NIH Record* 51:6.

[6] Ibid.

[7] Fernandez-Ballesteros, R. 2001. Cancer-prone personality, Type C. *International Encyclopedia of the Social and Behavioral Sciences*, 1439-43.

8 Spiegel, David, J. R. Bloom, H. C. Kraemer, and E. Gottheil. 1989. Effect of psychosocial treatment on survival of patients with metastatic breast cancer. *Lancet* 2(8668):888-91.

9 Dimeo, F. C. 2001. Effects of exercise on cancer-related fatigue. *Cancer* 92(6Suppl):1689-93.

10 Applebaum, A. B. and M. Brennan. 2009. Mental health and depression. *Older Adults with HIV: An In-Depth Examination of an Emerging Population* 27-34. Eds. M. Brennan, S. E. Karpiak, M. H. Cantor, and R. A. Shippy. New York: Nova Publishers.

11 Mednick, S. C., K. Nakayama, J. L. Cantero, M. Atieza, A. A. Levin, N. Pathak, and R. Stickgold. 2002. The restorative effect of naps on perceptual deterioration. *Nature Neuroscience* 5(7):677-81.

12 Stanhope, K. L., J. M. Schwartz, N. L. Keim, S. C. Griffen, A. A. Bremer, J. L. Graham, B. Hatcher, et al. 2009. Consuming fructose-sweetened beverages increases adiposity and lipids and decreases insulin sensitivity in overweight/obese humans. *Journal of Clinical Investigation* 119(5):1322-34.

13 Gill, D. J., K. M. Tham, J. Chia, S. C. Wang, C. Steentoft, H. Clausen, E. A. Bard-Chapeau, and F. A. Bard. 2013. Initiation of GalNAc-type O-glycosylation in the endoplasmic reticulum promotes cancer cell invasiveness. *Proceedings of the National Academy of Sciences* 110(34):E3152-61.

14 Adapted from Holmes-Rahe Social Readjustment Rating Scale. 1967. *Journal of Psychosomatic Research* 11(2): 213-8.

15 Blumenthal, J. A., M. A. Babyak, K. A. Moore, W. E. Craighead, S. Herman, P. Khatri, R. Waugh, et al. 1999. Effects of exercise training on older patients with major depression. *Archives of Internal Medicine* 159(19):2349-56.

16 Fleming, R., A. Baum, M. M. Gisriel, and R. J. Gatchel. 1982. Mediating influences of social support on stress at Three Mile Island. *Journal of Human Stress* 8(3):14-22.

17 Sonntag W. E., C. Lynch, P. Thornton, A. Khan, S. Bennett, and R. Ingram. 2000. The effects of growth hormone and IGF-1 deficiency on cerebrovascular and brain aging. *Journal of Anatomy* 197(4):575-85.

[18] Shapiro, A. C., T. T. Rogers, N. I. Cordova, N. B. Turk-Browne, and M. M. Botvinick. 2013. Neural representation of events arise from temporal community structure. *Nature Neuroscience* 16(4):486-92.

[19] Kiecolt-Glaser, J. K., R. Glaser, D. Williger, J. Stout, G. Messick, S. Sheppard, D. Ricker, et al. 1985. Psychosocial enhancement of immunocompetence in a geriatric population. *Health Psychology* 4(1):25-41.

[20] Desbordes, G., L. T. Negi, T. W. Pace, B. A. Wallace, C. L. Raison, and E. L. Schwartz 2012. Effects of mindful-attention and compassion meditation training on amygdala response to emotional stimuli in an ordinary, non-meditative state. *Frontiers of Human Neuroscience* 10:3389.

[21] Borysenko, J. 2007. *Minding the Body, Mending the Mind.* Boston: DaCapo Press.

[22] Zakowski, S., M. H. Hall, and A. Baum. 1992. Stress, stress management, and the immune system. *Applied and Preventive Psychology* 1(1):1-13.

[23] McKinney, C. H., M. H. Antoni, M. Kumar, F. C. Tims, and P. M. McCabe. 1997. Effects of guided imagery and music (GIM) therapy on mood and cortisol in healthy adults. *Health Psychology* 16(4):390-400.

[24] Lengacher, C. A., M. P. Bennett, L. Gonzalez, D. Gilvary, E. C. Cox, A. Cantor, P.B. Jacobsen, C Yang, and J. Djeu. 2008. Immune responses to guided imagery during breast cancer treatment. *Biological Research for Nursing* 9(3):205-14.

[25] Eremin, O., M. B. Walker, E. Simpson, S. D. Heys, A. K. Ah-See, A. W. Hutcheon, K. N. Ogston, T. K. Sarkar, A. Segar, and L. G. Walker. 2009. Immuno-modulatory effects of relaxation training and guided imagery in women with locally advanced breast cancer undergoing multimodality therapy: A randomized controlled trial. *The Breast* 18(1):17-25.

[26] Cohen, L., P. A. Parker, L. Vence, C. Savary, D. Kentor, C. Pettaway, R. Babaian, et al. 2011. Presurgical stress management improves postoperative immune function in men with prostate cancer undergoing radical prostatectomy. *Psychosomatic Medicine* 73(3):218-25.

27 Vancampfort, D., C. U. Correll, T. W. Scheewe, M. Probst, A. De Herdt, J. Knapen, and M. De Hert. 2013. Progressive muscle relaxation in persons with schizophrenia: A systematic review of randomized controlled trials. *Clinical Rehabilitaion* 27(4):291-8.

28 Nationwide poll taken April 20-22, 1998, and reported on CBS news April 29, 1998.

29 Koenig, H. G., J. C. Hays, D. B. Larson, L. K. George, H. J. Cohen, M. E. McCullough, K. G. Meador, and D. G. Blazer. 1999. Does religious attendance prolong survival? A six-year follow-up study of 3,968 older adults. *Journals of Gerontology Series A: Biological Sciences and Medical Sciences* 54(A):M370-6.

30 Koenig, H. G., L. K. George, and B. L. Peterson. 1998. Religiosity and remission of depression in medically ill older adults. *The American Journal of Psychiatry* 155(4):536-42.

31 Report from BBC News. Nov. 12, 1999. *Praying Aids Mental Health.*

32 Findings presented at the 116th Annual Meeting of the American Academy of Ophthalmology, Oct. 9-12, 2012.

References

CHAPTER ONE: **The Brain: Where It All Starts**

Ader, R. 1981. *Psychoneuroimmunology*. San Diego: Academic Press.

Ader, R., N. Cohen, and D. Felten. 1995.
Psychoneuroimmunology: Interactions between the nervous
system and immune system. *Lancet* 345(8942):99-103.

Adler, N. and K. Matthews. 1994. Health psychology: Why do
some people get sick and some stay well? *Annual Review of
Psychology* 45:229-59.

Anisman, H., J. Griffiths, K. Matheson, A. V. Ravindran, and Z.
Merali. 2001. Posttraumatic stress symptoms and salivary
cortisol levels. *American Journal of Psychiatry* 158(9):1509-11.

Astin, J. A., S. L. Shapiro, D. M. Eisenberg, and K. L. Forys. 2003.
Mind-body medicine: State of the science, implications
for practice. *Journal of the American Board of Family Practice*
16(2):131-47.

Benson, H. 1979. *The Mind-Body Effect*. New York: Simon &
Schuster.

Benson, H. 1996. *Timeless Healing: The Power and Biology of Belief*.
New York: Scribner & Sons.

Cotman, C. W., R. E. Brinton, A. Galaburda, B. McEwen, and
D. M. Schnieder, eds.. 1987. *The Neuro-Immune-Endocrine
Connection*. New York: Raven Press.

Cunningham, A. 2001. Ivan Pavlov and the conditioning of physiological responses. *Advances in Mind Body Medicine* 17(1):7-8.

DeCuevas, J. 1994. Mind, Brain and Behavior. *Harvard Magazine* 97(2): 36-43.

Gordon, J. S. 1996. *Manifesto for a New Medicine: Your Guide to Healing Partnerships and the Wise Use of Alternative Therapies.* Reading, Mass.: Addison-Wesley.

Kendler, K. S. 2001. A psychiatric dialogue on the mind-body problem. *American Journal of Psychiatry* 158(7):989-1000.

Kropiunigg, U. 1993. Basics in psychoneuroimmunology. *Annals of Medicine* 25(5):473-9.

Larson, M. R., R. Ader, and J. A. Moynihan. 2001. Heart rate, neuroendocrine, and immunological reactivity in response to an acute laboratory stressor. *Psychosomatic Medicine*, 63(3):493-501.

Marsh, J. A. and M. D. Kendall. 1996. *The Physiology of Immunity.* New York: CRC Press.

Martin, P. 1998. *The Healing Mind: The Vital Links Between Brain and Behavior, Immunity and Disease.* New York: St. Martin's Press.

Mehl-Madrona, L. 2001. Placebos and their effectiveness. *Advances in Mind Body Medicine* 17(1):17-8.

Morgan, C. A., S. Wang, A Rasmusson, G. Hazlett, G. Anderson, and D. S. Charney. 2001. Relationship among plasma cortisol, catecholamines, neuropeptide Y, and human performance during exposure to uncontrollable stress. *Psychosomatic Medicine* 63(3):412-22.

Ogden, T. H. 2001. Re-minding the body. *American Journal of Psychotherapy* 55(1):92-104.

Ornstein, R. and D. Sobel. 1987. *The Healing Brain.* New York: Simon & Schuster.

Pelletier, K. R. 1977. *Mind as Healer, Mind as Slayer.* New York: Delta.

Pelletier, K. R. 1994. *Sound Mind, Sound Body: A New Model for Lifelong Health.* New York: Simon & Schuster.

Sapolsky, R. M. 1994. *Why Zebras Don't Get Ulcers: A Guide to Stress, Stress Related Diseases, and Coping.* New York: W. H. Freeman.

Sapolsky, R. M. 2000. Glucocorticoids and hippocampal atrophy in neuropsychiatric disorders. *Archives of General Psychiatry* 57(10):925-35.

Schimmel, P. 2001. Mind over matter? Philosophical aspects of the mind-brain problem. *Australian and New Zealand Journal of Psychiatry* 35(4):481-7.

Seiden, O. J. 1998. *5-HTP: The Serotonin Connection.* Rocklin, Calif.: Prima Health.

Sluiter, J. K., M. H. Frings-Dresen, A. J. van der Beek, and T. F. Meijman. 2001. The relation between work-induced neuroendocrine reactivity and recovery, subjective need for recovery, and health status. *Journal of Psychosomatic Research* 50(1):29-37.

Solomon, G. F. and A. A. Amkraut. 1981. Psychoneuroendocrinological effects on the immune response. *Annual Review of Microbiology* 35:155-84.

Stefano, G. B., G. L. Fricchione, B. T. Slingsby, and H. Benson. 2001. The placebo effect and relaxation response: neural processes and their coupling to constitutive nitric oxide. *Brain Research* 35(1):1-19.

von Kanel, R., P. J. Mills, C. Fainman, and J. E. Dimsdale. 2001. Effects of psychological stress and psychiatric disorders on blood coagulation and fibrinolysis: A biobehavioral pathway to coronary artery disease? *Psychosomatic Medicine* 63(4): 531-44.

CHAPTER TWO: **Why and How We Get Sick**

Adler, N. and K. Matthews. 1994. Health psychology: Why do some people get sick and some stay well? *Annual Review of Psychology* 45:229-59.

Anderson, D. E. 1984. Interactions of stress, salt, and blood pressure. *Annual Review of Physiology* 46:143-53.

Arking, R. 1991. *Biology of Aging: Observations and Principles.* Englewood Cliffs, N.J: Prentice Hall.

Buckingham, J. C., G. E. Gillies, and A. M. Cowell, eds. 1999. *Stress, Stress Hormones, and the Immune System*. New York: John Wiley and Sons.

Cherniske, S. 1996. *The DHEA Breakthrough*. New York: Ballantine Books.

Cohen, S. and T. Herbert. 1996. Health psychology: Psychologic factors and physical disease from the perspective of human psychoneuroimmunology. *Annual Review of Psychology*, 47:113-42.

Cohen, S., D.A. Tyrrell, and A. P. Smith. 1991. Psychological stress and susceptibility to the common cold. *New England Journal of Medicine* 325(9):606-12.

Cohen, S., D. Janicki-Deverts, and G. E. Miller. 2007. Psychological stress and disease (HIV/AIDS). *Journal of the American Medical Association* 298(14):1685-7.

Dantzer, R. and K. W. Kelley. 1989. Stress and immunity: An integrated view of relationships between the brain and the immune system. *Life Science* 44(26):1995-2008.

Evans, R., M. L. Barer, and T. R. Marmor, eds.. 1994. *Why Are Some People Healthy and Others Not?* New York: Aldine De Gruyter.

Everson, S., G. A. Kaplan, D. E. Goldberg, T. A. Lakka, J. Sivenius, and J. T. Salonen. 1999. Anger expression and incident stroke: Prospective evidence from the Kuopio ischemic heart disease study. *Stroke* 30(13):523-8.

Eysenck, H. J. 1988. Personality, stress, and cancer: Prediction and prophylaxis. *British Journal of Medical Psychology* 61(Pt1):57-75.

Finch, C. E. 1990. *Longevity, Senescence, and the Genome*. Chicago: University of Chicago Press.

Freier, S. 1990. *The Neuroendocrine-Immune Network*. Boca Raton, Fla.: CRC Press.

George, M. S., T. A. Ketter, P. I. Parekh, B. Horwitz, P. Herscovitch, and R. M. Post. 1995. Brain activity during transient sadness and happiness in healthy women. *American Journal of Psychiatry* 152(13):341-57.

Goliszek, A. G. 1983. *Effects of physical and emotional stress on cholesterol and LDL levels.* Ph.D. Dissertation, Utah State University.

Goliszek, A. G., G. E. Crawford, H. S. Lawrence, J. Bennett, F. Williams, and S. L. Hurley. 1996. Effects of prepubertal stress on subsequent ACTH response to novel stress and CRH in male vs. female rats. *Stress Medicine* 12(3):199-204.

Guyton, A. C. and J. E. Hall. 1997. *Human Physiology and Mechanisms of Disease.* New York: W. B. Saunders Co..

Herbert, T. B. and S. Cohen. 1993. Stress and immunity in humans: A meta-analytic review. *Psychosomatic Medicine* 55(4):364-79.

Jemmott, J. B. and S. E. Locke. 1984. Psychosocial factors and human susceptibility to infectious diseases: How much do we know? *Psychology Bulletin* 95(1):78-108.

Jiang, W., M. Babyak, D. S. Krantz, R. A. Waugh, R. E. Coleman, M. M. Hanson, D. J. Frid, et al. 1996. Mental stress-induced myocardial ischemia and cardiac events. *Journal of the American Medical Association* 275(21):1651-6.

Keynes, W. M. 1994. Medical response to mental stress. *Journal of the Royal Society of Medicine* 87(9):536-9.

Kiecolt-Glaser, J. K. and R. Glaser. 1991. *Stress and immune function in humans.* In *Psychoneuroimmunology,.* 2nd ed, eds. R. Ader, D. Felten, and N. Cohen. San Diego: Academic Press.

Kiecolt-Glaser, J.K., J. T. Cacioppo, W. B. Malarkey, and R. Glaser. 1992. Acute psychological stressors and short-term immune changes: what, why, for whom, and to what extent? *Psychosomatic Medicine* 54(6):680-5.

Kiecolt-Glaser, J. K. and R. Glaser. 1995. Psychoneuroimmunology and health consequences: Data and shared mechanisms. *Psychosomatic Medicine* 57(3):269-74.

Krantz, D. S., W. J. Kop, H. T. Santiago, and J. S. Gottdiener. 1996. Mental stress as a trigger for myocardial ischemia and infarction. *Cardiology Clinics* 14(2):271-87.

Marcus, M. B. 2007. Graying of America takes mental toll, too. *USA Today*, July 31, 2006.

Mayou, R. and M. Sharpe. 1995. Diagnosis, disease, and illness. *Quarterly Journal of Medicine* 88(11):827-31.

Morimoto, R. I. 2006. Stress, aging, and neurodegenerative disease. *New England Journal of Medicine* 355(21):2254-5.

Pasnau, R. O. 1984. Psychiatric considerations in coronary artery disease. *Bulletin of Menninger Clinic* 48(3):209-20.

Pereira, D. B., D. H. Antoni, A. Danielson, T. Simon, J. Efantis-Potter, C. S. Cramer, and R. E. Durán, et al. 2003. Stress as a predictor of symptomatic genital herpes virus recurrence in women with human immunodeficiency virus. *Journal of Psychosomatic Research* 54(3):237-44.

Rabin, B. S., S. Cohen, R. Ganguli, D. T. Lysle, and J. E. Cunnick. 1989. Bidirectional interaction between the central nervous system and the immune system. *Critical Review of Immunology* 9(4):279-312.

Rahe, R. H. 1988. Anxiety and physical illness. *Journal of Clinical Psychiatry* 49 Suppl:26-9.

Sapolsky, R. M. 1994. *Why Zebras Don't Get Ulcers: A Guide to Stress, Stress Related Diseases, and Coping.* New York: W.H. Freeman.

Schneiderman, N. 1999. Behavioral medicine and the management of HIV/AIDS. *International Journal of Behavioral Medicine* 6(1):3-12.

Seeman, T. E. and B. S. McEwen. 1996. Impact of social environment characteristics on neuroendocrine regulation. *Psychosomatic Medicine* 58(5):459-71.

Selye, H. 1946. The General Adaptation Syndrome and the diseases of adaptation. *Journal of Clinical Endocrinology* 6(2):117-230.

Selye, H. 1974. *Stress Without Distress.* New York: Dutton.

Selye, H. 1978. *The Stress of Life,* rev. ed.. New York: McGraw-Hill.

Siltanen, P. 1987. Stress, coronary disease, and coronary death. *Annals of Clinical Research* 19(2):96-103.

Somervell, P. D., B. H. Kaplan, G. Heiss, H. A. Tyroler, D. G. Kleinbaum, and P A. Obrist. 1989. Psychological distress as a predictor of mortality. *American Journal of Epidemiology* 130(5):1013-23.

Spangelo, B. L. 1995. The thymic-endocrine connection. *Journal of Endocrinology* 147(1):5-10.

Stone, A. A. and D. H. Bovbjerg. 1994. Stress and humoral immunity. *Advances in Neuroimmunology* 4(1):49-56.

Stone, A. A. and J. E. Broderick. 2001. Colds and the stress-illness connection. *Advances in Mind Body Medicine* 17(1):41-3.

United Nations. 2002. *Report of the Second World Assembly on Aging.* Presented in Madrid, Spain, April 8-12.

Vedhara, K. and M. Irwin, eds. 2005. *Human Psychoneuroimmunology.* Oxford, U.K.: OxZford University Press.

Williams, R. B. 2001. Hostility and heart disease. *Advances in Mind Body Medicine* 17(1):52-5.

CHAPTER THREE: **Using the Mind-Body Connection to Prevent Disease**

Adams, A. K., E. O. Wermuth, and P. E. McBride. 1999. Antioxidant vitamins and the prevention of coronary artery disease. *American Family Physician* 60(3):895-904.

Alessio, H. M., and E. R. Blasi. 1997. Physical activity as a natural antioxidant booster and its effects on a healthy life span. *Research Quarterly for Exercise and Sport* 68(4):292-302.

Anderson, B. L., W. B. Farrar, D. Golden-Kreutz, L. A. Kutz, R. MacCallum, M. E. Courtney, and R. Glaser. 1998. Stress and immune responses after surgical treatment for regional breast cancer. *Journal of the National Cancer Institute* 90(1):30-6.

Berczi, I., and J. Szelenyi, eds. 1994. Advances in psycho-neuroimmunology. In *Hans Selye Symposia on Neuroendocrinology and Stress, vol. 3.* New York: Plenum.

Borysenko, J. 1987. *Minding the Body, Mending the Mind.* Boston: Addison-Wesley.

Buckingham, J. C. 1996. Stress and the neuroendocrine-immune axis: the pivotal role of glucocorticoids and lipocortin 1. *British Journal of Pharmacology* 118(1):1-19.

Cohen, S. and T. B. Herbet. 1996. Health psychology: psychologic factors and physical disease from the perspective of human psychoneuroimmunology. *Annual Review of Psychology* 47:113-42.

Cousins, N. 1979. *Anatomy of an Illness as Perceived by the Patient: Reflections on Healing and Regeneration*. New York: Bantam Books.

Danenberg, H. D., A. Ben-Yehuda, Z. Zakay-Rones, and G. Friedman. 1995. Dehydroepiandrosterone (DHEA) treatment reverses the impaired immune response of old mice to influenza vaccination and protects from influenza infection. *Vaccine* 13(15):1445-8.

Fawzy, F. I., N. W. Fawzy, C. S. Hyun, R. Elashoff, D. Guthrie, J. L. Fahey, and D. L. Morton. 1993. Malignant melanoma: Effects of an early structured psychiatric intervention, coping, and affective state on recurrence and survival six years later. *Archives of General Psychiatry* 50(9):681-9.

Fitzgerald, L. 1988. Exercise and the immune system. *Immunology Today* 9(11)-337-9.

Glassman, J. 1983. *The Cancer Survivors: And How They Did It*. New York: Doubleday.

Hauri, P. and S. Linde. 1996. *No More Sleepless Nights*. Somerset, N. J.: John Wiley and Sons.

Hobson, J. A. 1989. *Sleep*. New York: Scientific American Library.

Hughes, M. 1989. *Body Clock: The Effects of Time on Human Health*. London: Weidenfeld and Nicolson.

Jezova, D., I. Skultetyova, D. I. Tokarev, P. Bakos, and M. Vigas. 1995. Vasopressin and oxytocin in stress. *Annals of the New York Academy of Science* 771:192-203.

Kate, N. T. 1994. To reduce stress, hit the hay. *American Demographics* 16(9):14-15.

Morin, C. M. 1996. *Relief From Insomnia*. New York: Doubleday.

Null, G. 1999. *Get Healthy Now: A Complete Guide to Prevention, Treatment, and Healthy Living*. New York: Seven Stories Press.

Ornish, D. 1998. *Love and Survival: The Scientific Basis for the Healing Power of Intimacy*. New York: Harper Collins.

Peale, N. V. 1959. *The Amazing Results of Positive Thinking*. New York: Fawcett Columbine.

Rabin, B. S., S. Cohen, R. Ganguli, D. T. Lysle, and J. E. Cunnick. 1989. Bidirectional interaction between the central nervous system and immune system. *Critical Review of Immunology* 9(4):279-312.

Schwartz, A. G., L. Pashko, and J. M. Whitcomb. 1986. Inhibition of tumor development by dehydroepiandrosterone and other related steroids. *Toxicology and Pathology* 14(3):357-62.

Siegel, B. S. 1986. *Love, Medicine and Miracles: Lessons Learned about Self-Healing from a Surgeon's Experience with Exceptional Patients.*. New York: Harper and Row.

Somervell, P. D., B. H. Kaplan, G. Heiss, H. A. Tyroler, D. G. Kleinbaum, and P. A. Obrist. 1989. Psychological distress as a predictor of mortality. *American Journal of Epidemiology* 130(5):1013-23.

Spiegel, D., J. R. Bloom, H. C. Kraemer, and E. Gottheil. 1989. Effect of psychosocial treatment on survival of patients with metastatic breast cancer. *The Lancet* 2(8668):888-91.

Spiegel, K. 1999. Impact of sleep debt on metabolic and endocrine function. *The Lancet* 354(9188):1435-9.

Wilder, R. L. 1995. Neuroendocrine-immune system interactions and autoimmunity. *Annual Review of Immunology* 13:307-38.

Winawer, S. J. and M. Shike. 1994. *Cancer Free: The Comprehensive Cancer Prevention Program*. New York: Simon & Schuster.

CHAPTER FOUR: **Conditioning the Brain to Prevent Illness**

Aguilera, G. 1994. Regulation of pituitary ACTH release during chronic stress. *Frontiers in Neuroendocrinology* 15(4):321-50.

Armario, A., A. Lopez-Calderone, T. Jolin, and J. Balasch. 1986. Response of anterior pituitary hormones to chronic stress: The specificity of adaptation. *Neuroscience and Behavior Review* 10(3):245-50.

Bell, C., J. Abrams, and D. Nutt. 2001. Tryptophan depletion and its implications for psychiatry. *British Journal of Psychiatry* 178:399-405.

Benson, H. 1975. *The Relaxation Response: How to Harness the Healing Power of Your Personal Beliefs*. New York: William Morrow.

Benson, H. 1984. *Beyond the Relaxation Response*. New York: Times Books.

Davis, M., E. R. Eshelman, and M. McKay. 1995. *The Relaxation and Stress Reduction Workbook*. New York: MJF Books.

Fitzgerald, L. 1988. Exercise and the immune system. *Immunology Today* 9(11):337-9.

Girdano, D. A., G. S. Everly, and D. E. Dusek. 1993. *Controlling Stress and Tension: A Holistic Approach*. Englewood Cliffs, N. J.: Prentice Hall.

Glaser, R. and J. K. Kiecolt-Glaser. 1994. *Handbook of Stress and Immunity*. San Diego: Academic Press.

Goliszek, A. 1987. *Breaking the Stress Habit: A Modern Guide to One-Minute Stress Management*. Winston-Salem, N. C.: Carolina Press.

Goliszek, A. 1992. *Sixty-Second Stress Management: The Quickest Way to Relax and Ease Anxiety*. Far Hills, N. J.: New Horizon Press.

Goodloe, A., J. Bensahel and J. Kelly. 1984. *Managing Yourself: How to Control Emotion, Stress and Time*. New York: Franklin Watts.

Holmes, T. H. and R. H. Rahe. 1968. The social readjustment rating scale. *Journal of Psychosomatic Research* 11(2):213-8.

Kinney, J. M. and H. N. Tucker. 1997. *Physiology, Stress, and Malnutrition: Functional Correlates, Nutritional Intervention*. New York: Lippincott, Williams & Wilkins.

Levenstein, S., A. Ackerman, J. K. Kiecolt-Glaser, and A. Dubois. 1999. Stress and peptic ulcer disease. *Journal of the American Medical Association* 281(1):10-1.

Maltz, M. and B. Sommer. 1993. *Psycho-Cybernetics*. New York: MJF Books

McEwen, B. S. 1997. Possible mechanisms for atrophy of the human hippocampus. *Molecular Psychiatry* 2(3):255-62.

McEwen, B. S. 1998. Protective and damaging effects of stress mediators. *New England Journal of Medicine*, 338(3): 171-9.

Newcomer, J. W., G. Selke, A. K. Melson, T. Hershey, S. Craft, K. Richards, and A. L. Alderson. 1999. Decreased memory performance in healthy humans induced by stress-level cortisol treatment. *Archives of General Psychiatry* 56(6): 527-33.

Potter, B. A. 1987. *Preventing Job Burnout: Transforming Work Pressures into Productivity*. Los Altos, Calif.: Crisp Publications.

Rahe, R. H. and R. J. Arthur. 1978. Life change and illness studies: Past history and future directions. *Journal of Human Stress* 4(1):3-15.

Sapolsky, R. M. 1994. *Why Zebras Don't Get Ulcers: A Guide to Stress, Stress Related Diseases, and Coping.* New York: W. H. Freeman.

Siegman, A. W., S. T. Townsend, A. C. Civelek, and R. S. Blumenthal. 2000. Antagonistic behavior, dominance, hostility, and coronary heart disease. *Psychosomatic Medicine* 62(2):248-57.

Stine, G. L. 1999. *AIDS Update.* Upper Saddle River, N. J.: Prentice Hall.

Tubesing, N. L. and D. A. Tubesing. 1990. *Structured Exercises in Stress Management: A Whole Person Handbook for Trainers, Educators, and Group Leaders.* Duluth, Minn.: Whole Person Press.

Wolff, A. C. and P. A. Ratner. 1999. Stress, social support, and sense of coherence. *West Journal of Nursing Research* 21(2): 182-97.

CHAPTER FIVE: **Stress, Mental Health, and the Mind-Body Connection**

Abush, R. and E. J. Burkhead. 1984. Job stress in midlife working women: Relationships among personality type, job characteristics, and job tensions. *Journal of Counseling Psychology* 31(1):36-44.

Cohen, S., D. A. Tyrrell, and A. P. Smith. 1991. Psychological stress and susceptibility to the common cold. *New England Journal of Medicine* 325(9):606-12.

Cummings, N. and J. L. Cummings. 2000. *The Essence of Psychotherapy: Reinventing the Art in the New Era of Data..* San Diego: Academic Press.

Evans, D. L. 1989. Immune correlates of stress and depression. *Psychopharmacology Bulletin* 25(3):319-24.

Hall, M., D. J. Buysse, P. D. Nowell, E. A. Nofzinger, P. Houck, C. F. Reynolds III, and D. J. Kupfer. 2000. Symptoms of stress and depression as correlates of sleep in primary insomnia. *Psychosomatic Medicine* 62(2):227-30.

Irie, M., S. Asami, S. Nagata, M. Ikeda, M. Miyata, and H. Kasai. 2001. Psychosocial factors as a potential trigger of oxidative DNA damage in human leukocytes. *Japanese Journal of Cancer Research* 92(3):367-76.

Kendler, K. S., L. M. Karkowski, and C. A. Prescott. 1999. Causal relationship between stressful life events and the onset of major depression. *American Journal of Psychiatry* 156(6): 837-41.

Kleinknecht, R. A. 1991. *Mastering Anxiety: The Nature and Treatment of Anxious Conditions.* New York: Insight Books.

Lark, S. M. 1996. *Anxiety and Stress.* Berkeley, Calif.: Celestial Arts.

Lazarus, A. A. 1997. *The 60-Second Shrink.* New York: Barnes and Noble Books.

Levenstein, S., M. W. Smith, and G. A. Kaplan. 2001. Psychosocial predictors of hypertension in men and women. *Archives of Internal Medicine* 161(10):1341-6.

Lewy, A. J., B. J. Lefler, J. S. Emens, and V. K. Bauer. 2006. The circadian basis of winter depression. *Proceedings of the National Academy of Sciences* 103(19):7414-9.

Maciejewski, P. K. and C. M. Mazure. 2000. Stressful life events and depression. *American Journal of Psychiatry* 157(8):1344-5.

Mazure, C. M., M. L. Bruce, P. K. Maciejewski, and S. C. Jacobs. 2000. Adverse life events and cognitive-personality characteristics in the prediction of major depression and antidepressant responses. *American Journal of Psychiatry* 157(6):896-903.

Nemeroff, M. D., D. L. Musselman, and D. L. Evans. 1998. Depression and cardiac disease. *Depression and Anxiety* 8(Suppl1):71-9.

Nicoloff, G. and T. Schwenk. 1995. Using exercise to ward off depression. *Physician and Sports Medicine* 23(9):44-56.

Norden, M. J. 1995. *Beyond Prozac: Brain-Toxic Lifestyles, Natural Antidotes, and New Generation Antidepressants.* New York: Harper Collins.

North, C. S., S. J. Nixon, S. Shariat, S. Mallonee, J. C. McMillen, E. L. Sptiznagel, and E. M. Smith. 1999. Psychiatric disorders among survivors of the Oklahoma City bombing. *Journal of the American Medical Association* 282(8):755-62.

O'Leary, A. 1990. Stress, emotion, and human immune function. *Psychology Bulletin* 108(3):363-82.

Papolos, D., and J. Papalos. 1987. *Overcoming Depression.* Mount Vernon, N. Y.: Consumers Union.

Pickering, T. G. 2001. Mental stress as a causal factor in the development of hypertension and cardiovascular disease. *Current Hypertension Reports* 3(3):249-54.

Schleifer, S. J., S. E. Keller, M. Camerino, J. C. Thornton, and M. Stein. 1983. Suppression of lymphocyte stimulation following bereavement. *Journal of the American Medical Association* 250(3):374-7.

Schleifer, S.J., S. E. Keller, S. G. Siris, K. L. Davis, and M. Stein. 1985. Depression and immunity: Lymphocyte function in ambulatory depressed patients, hospitalized schizophrenic patients, and patients hospitalized for herniorrhaphy. *Archives of General Psychiatry* 42(2):129-33.

Zohman, B. L. 1973. Emotional factors in coronary disease. *Geriatrics* 28(2):110-9.

CHAPTER SIX: **Aging and the Mind-Body Connection**

Ardelt, M. 1997. Wisdom and life satisfaction in old age. *Journal of Gerontology* 52(1):15-27.

Arking, R. 1991. *Biology of Aging: Observations and Principles.* Englewood Cliffs, N. J.: Prentice Hall.

Austad, S. N. 1997. *Why We Age: What Science is Discovering about the Body's Journey through Life.* Somerset, N. J.: John Wiley and Sons.

Bernarducci, M. P. and N. J. Owens. 1996. Is there a fountain of youth? A review of current life extension strategies. *Pharmacotherapy* 16(2):183-200.

Bloom, F. E., A. Lazerson, and L. Hofstadter. 1985. *Brain, Mind, and Behavior.* New York: W. H. Freeman and Co.

Bock, S. J. 1995. *Stay Young the Melatonin Way: The Natural Plan for Better Sleep, Better Sex and Longer Life.* New York: Dutton.

Bourne, E. J. 2000. *The Anxiety and Phobia Workbook.* Oakland, Calif.: New Harbinger Publications.

Carper, J. 1995. *Stop Aging Now! The Ultimate Plan for Staying Young and Reversing the Aging Process*. New York: Harper Collins.

Clarkson-Smith, L. and A. A. Hartley. 1989. Relationship between physical exercise and cognitive abilities in older adults. *Psychology and Aging* 4(2):183-9.

Cohen, G. D. 1988. *The Brain in Human Aging*. New York: Springer Publishing Co.

Cohen, H. J. 2000. *Taking Care After 50: A Self-care Guide for Seniors*. New York: Three Rivers Press.

Cooper, E. L. 1984. *Stress, Immunity and Aging*. New York: Marcel Dekker.

Davison, A. N. 1987. Pathophysiology of aging brain. *Gerontology* 33(3-4):129-35.

Dollemore, D. and C. Raymond. 1997. *Disease Free at 60-plus: Hundreds of Life-preserving Tips and Techniques to Defy Heart Trouble, Cancer, and Stroke*. Emmaus, Pa.: Rodale Press.

Finch, C. E. and E. L. Schneider. 1985. *Handbook of the Biology of Aging*. New York: Van Nostrand-Reinhold.

Finch, C. E. 1990. *Longevity, Senescence, and the Genome*. Chicago: University of Chicago Press.

Goldman, R., R. Klatz, and L. Berger. 1999. *Brain Fitness: Anti-Aging Strategies for Achieving Super Mind Power*. New York: Doubleday.

Glass, T., C. M. de Leon, R. A. Marottoli, and L. F. Berkman. 1999. Population-based study of social and productive activities as predictors of survival among elderly Americans. *British Medical Journal* 319(7208):478-83.

Hanner, I., F. Erkeller-Yuksel, P. Lydyard, V. Deneys, and M. De Bruyere. 1992. Lymphocyte populations as a function of age. *Immunology Today* 13(6):215-8.

Hayflick, L. 1994. *How and Why We Age*. New York: Ballantine Books.

Jarvik, L. F. 1988. Aging of the brain: How can we prevent it? *The Gerontologist* 28(6):739-47.

Khalsa, D. S. 1997. *Brain Longevity:* The Breakthrough Medical Program that Improves Your Mind and Memory. New York: Warner Books.

Kling, K. C., M. M. Seltzer, and C. D. Ryff. 1997. Distinctive late-life challenges: Implications for coping and well-being. *Psychology and Aging* 12(2):288-95.

Kraaij, V. and E. J. de Wilde. 2001. Negative life events and depressive symptoms in the elderly: A life span perspective. *Aging and Mental Health* 5(1):84-91.

Ljungquist, B. and G. Sundstrom. 1996. Health and social networks as predictors of survival in old age. *Scandinavian Journal of Social Medicine* 24(2):90-101.

National Institute on Aging. 1996. *In Search of the Secrets of Aging*. Bethesda, Md.: National Institutes of Health.

Paster, Z. 2001. *The Longevity Code: Your Personal Prescription for a Longer, Sweeter Life*. New York: Clarkson Potter.

Pearson, D. and S. Shaw. 1982. *Life Extension: A Practical Scientific Approach*. New York: Warner Books.

Rodin, J. 1986. Aging and health: Effects of the sense of control. *Science* 233(4770):1271-6.

Rowe, J. W. and R. L. Kahn. 1998. *Successful Aging*. New York: Pantheon.

Ryff, C. D. 1995. Psychological well-being in adult life. *Current Directions in Psychological Science* 4(4):99-104.

Sapolski, R. M. 1992. Stress and neuroendocrine changes during aging. *Generations* 16(4):35-38.

Scheller, M. D. 1992. *Growing Older, Feeling Better*. Palo Alto, Calif.: Bull Publishing

Sears, B. 1999. *The Anti-Aging Zone*. New York: Regan Books.

Vlassara, C. A. and M. Brownlee. 1987. Glucose and aging. *Scientific American* 256(5):90-6.

Walters, R. 1993. *Options: The Alternative Cancer Therapy Book*. Garden City Park, N. Y.: Avery Publishing Group.

CHAPTER SEVEN: Meditation

Balducci, L. and R. Meyer. 2001. Spirituality and medicine: A proposal. *Cancer Control* 8(4):368-76.

Benson, H. 1975. *The Relaxation Response*. New York: William Morrow.

Benson, H. 1984. *Beyond the Relaxation Response: How to Harness the Healing Power of Your Personal Beliefs*. New York: Times Books.

Benson, H. 1996. *Timeless Healing: The Power and Biology of Belief*. New York: Scribner.

Bodey, G. P. 2001. Physicians and patient spirituality. *Annals of Internal Medicine* 135(3):220.

Dilorenzo, P., R. Johnson, and M. Bussey. 2001. The role of spirituality in the recovery process. *Child Welfare* 80(2): 257-73.

Dossey, L. 1993. *Healing Words: The Power of Prayer and the Practice of Medicine*. New York: HarperCollins.

Dossey, L. 1999. Do religion and spirituality matter in health? A response to the recent article in *The Lancet*. *Alternative Therapies in Health and Medicine*, 5(3):16-8.

Dunkin, A., and G. Smith, eds. 1993. Meditation, the new balm for corporate stress. *Business Week* May 9.

Ellison, C. G. 1991. Religious involvement and subjective well-being. *Journal of Health and Social Behavior* 32(1):80-99.

Fried, R. 1999. *Breathe Well, Be Well: A Program to Relieve Stress, Anxiety, Asthma, Hypertension, Migraine, and Other Disorders for Better Health*. Somerset, N. J.: John Wiley and Sons.

Hanh, T. N. 1976. *The Miracle of Mindfulness: A Manual on Meditation*. Boston: Beacon Press.

Harp, D. and N. Feldman. 1996. *The Three-Minute Meditator*. New York: MJF Books.

Hixson, K. A., H. W. Gruchow, and D. W. Morgan. 1998. The relation between religiosity, selected health behaviors, and blood pressure among adult females. *Preventive Medicine* 27(4):545-52.

Kaptchuk, T. and M. Croucher. 1987. *The Healing Arts: Exploring the Medical Ways of the World*. New York: Summit Books.

Keefer, L. and E. B. Blanchard. 2001. The effects of relaxation response meditation on the symptoms of irritable bowel syndrome: Results of a controlled treatment study. *Behavioral Research and Therapeutics* 39(7):801-11.

Koenig, H. G. 1999. *The Healing Power of Faith: Science Explores Medicine's Last Great Frontier*. New York: Simon and Schuster.

Koren, L. 1991. *Noise Reduction: A Ten-Minute Meditation for Quieting the Mind*. New York: St. Martin's Press.

Lawlor, J. 1993. Meditation "takes the edge off" at work. *USA Today* June 18.

McBride, J. L., G. Arthur, R. Brooks, and L. Pilkington. 1998. The relationship between a patient's spirituality and health experiences. *Family Medicine* 30(2):122-6.

Seligman, M. E. and M. Csikszentmihalyi. 2000. Positive psychology: An introduction. *American Psychologist* 55(1): 5-14.

Targ, R. and J. Katra. 1998. *Miracles of Mind: Exploring Nonlocal Consciousness and Spiritual Healing*. Novato, Calif.: New World Library.

Waldfogel, S. 1997. Spirituality in medicine. *Primary Care: Clinics in Office Practice* 24(4):963-76.

Zi, N. 1986. *The Art of Breathing*. New York: Bantam Books.

CHAPTER EIGHT: **Guided Imagery and Self-Healing**

Achterberg, J., B. M. Dossey, and L. Kolkmeier. 1994. *Rituals of Healing: Using Imagery for Health and Wellness*. New York: Bantam Doubleday Dell.

Bazzo, D. J. and R. A. Moeller. 1999. Imagine this! Infinite uses of guided imagery in women's health. *Journal of Holistic Nursing* 17(4):317-30.

Dahm, N. C. 2000. *Mind, Body, and Soul: A Guide to Living with Cancer*. Garden City, N. Y.: Taylor Hill Publishing.

Denning, M., and O. Phillips. 1984. *Practical Guide to Creative Visualization: Proven Techniques to Shape Your Destiny*. St. Paul, Minn.: Llewellyn Publications.

Epstein, G. 1989. *Healing Visualizations: Creating Health through Imagery*. New York: Bantam.

Fezler, W. D. 1989. *Creative Imagery: How to Visualize in All Five Senses.* . Upper Saddle River, N. J.: Prentice Hall.

Goliszek, A. 1987. *Breaking the Stress Habit: A Modern Guide to One-Minute Stress Management*. Winston-Salem, N. C.: Carolina Press.

Klaus, L., A. Beniaminovitz, L. Choi, F. Greenfield, G. C. Whitworth, M. C. Oz, and D. M. Mancini. 2000. Pilot study of guided imagery use in patients with severe heart failure. *American Journal of Cardiology* 86(1):101-4.

Langley, P. 1999. Guided imagery: A review of effectiveness in the care of children. *Paediatric Nursing* 11(3):18-21.

Lusk, J. T. 1992. *Thirty Scripts for Relaxation Imagery and Inner Healing*. Duluth, Minn.: Whole Person Associates.

Maack, C. and P. Nolan. 1999. The effects of guided imagery and music therapy on reported change in normal adults. *Journal of Music Therapy* 36(1):39-55.

Mannix, L. K., R. S. Chandurkar, L. A. Rybicki, D. L. Tusek, and G. D. Solomon. 1999. Effect of guided imagery on quality of life for patients with chronic tension-type headache. *Headache* 39(5):326-34.

Pettinati, P. M. 2001. Meditation, yoga, and guided imagery. *Nurse Clinician of North America* 36(1):47-56.

Rossman, M. L. 2000. *Guided Imagery for Self-Healing: An Essential Resource for Anyone Seeking Wellness*. Tiburon, Calif.: H. J. Kramer.

Shone, R. 1998. *Creative Visualization: Using Imagery and Imagination for Self-Transformation*. Rochester, Vt.: Destiny Books.

Siegel, B. S. 1986. *Love, Medicine, and Miracles: Lessons Learned about Self-Healing from a Surgeon's Experience with Exceptional Patients*. New York: Harper and Row.

Tusek, D. L. 1999. Guided imagery: A powerful tool to decrease length of stay, pain, anxiety, and narcotic consumption. *Journal of Invasive Cardiology* 11(4):265-7.

Walker, L. G., S. D. Heys, and O. Eremin. 1999. Surviving cancer: Do psychological factors count? *Journal of Psychosomatic Research* 47(6):497-503.

CHAPTER NINE: **Relaxation Exercises and Techniques**

Davis, M., E. R. Eshelman and M. McKay. 1995. *The Relaxation and Stress Reduction Workbook*. New York: MJF Books.

Epstein, R. 1998. *Stress Management and Relaxation Activities for Trainers*. New York: McGraw-Hill.

Evans, J. R. and A. Abarbanel. 1999. *Introduction to Quantitative EEG and Neurofeedback*. San Diego: Academic Press.

Gallagher-Mundy, C. 1995. *Relaxation: An Illustrated Program of Exercises, Techniques and Meditations*. Collingdale, Pa.: Diane Publishing.

Goliszek, A. 1987. *Breaking the Stress Habit: A Modern Guide to One-Minute Stress Management*. Winston-Salem, N. C.: Carolina Press.

Goliszek, A. 1992. *Sixty-Second Stress Management: The Quickest Way to Relax and Ease Anxiety*. Far Hills, N. J.: New Horizon Press.

Jacobson, E. 1938. *Progressive Relaxation: A Physiological and Clinical Investigation of Muscular States and Their Significance in Psychology and Medical Practice*. Chicago: University of Chicago Press.

Klarreich, S. H. 1990. *Work without Stress: A Practical Guide to Emotional and Physical Well-being on the Job*. New York: Brunner/Mazel Publishers.

Lowe, G., R. Bland, J. Greenman, N. Kirkpatrick, and G. Lowe. 2001. Progressive muscle relaxation and secretory immunoglobulin A. *Psychology Reports* 88(3pt1):912-4.

Peper, E., S. Ancoli-Israel, and M. Quinn. 1979. *Mind Body Integration: Essential Readings in Biofeedback*. New York: Plenum Publishing Co.

Robbins, J. 2000. *A Symphony in the Brain: The Evolution of the New Brain Wave Biofeedback*. New York: Grove Press.

Schwartz, M. S. and F. Andrasik. 1998. *Biofeedback: A Practitioner's Guide*. New York: The Guilford Press.

CHAPTER TEN: **Spirituality, Alternative Medicine, and Health**

Borland, D. 1982. *Homeopathy in Practice*. New Canaan, Conn.: Keats Publishing.

Castleman, M. 2000. *Blended Medicine: The Best Choices in Healing*. Emmaus, Pa.: Rodale Press.

Chappell, P. 1994. *Emotional Healing with Homeopathy: A Self-help Manual*. Rockport, Mass.: Element, Inc.

Flannery, G. R. 1997. Immunology: The immune system and beyond. In *The Web of Life,* eds. G. Padmanaban, M. Biswas, M. S. Shaila, and S. Vishveshwara. The Netherlands: Harwood Academic Publishers.

Gerber, R. 2000. *Vibrational Medicine for the Twenty-first Century: The Complete Guide to Energy Healing and Spiritual Transformation*. New York: William Morrow.

Goliszek, A. G. 1992. *Sixty-Second Stress Management: The Quickest Way to Relax and Ease Anxiety*. Far Hills, N. J.: New Horizon Press.

Lehrer, P. M. and R. L. Woolfolk. 1993. *Principles and Practice of Stress Management*. New York: Guilford Press.

Macrae, J. 1987. *Therapeutic Touch: A Practical Guide*. New York: Alfred A. Knopf.

McIntyre, A. 1996. *Flower Power: Flower Remedies for Healing Body and Soul through Herbalism, Homeopathy, Aromatherapy, and Flower Essence*. New York: Henry Holt and Company.

Murray, M. T. and J. E. Pizzorno. 1991. *Encyclopedia of Natural Medicine*. Rocklin, Calif.: Prima Publishing.

Norris, P. A. 1986. Biofeedback, voluntary control, and human potential. *Biofeedback and Self-Regulation* 11:1-20.

Rosenfeld, I. 1996. *Dr. Rosenfeld's Guide to Alternative Medicine: What Works, What Doesn't, and What's Right for You*. New York: Random House.

Shealy, C. N. 1995. *Miracles Do Happen: A Physician's Experience with Alternative Medicine*. Rockport, Mass.: Element Books.

Walters, R. 1993. *Options: The Alternative Cancer Therapy Book*. Garden City Park, N. Y. Avery Publishing Group.

Weil, A. 1990. *Natural Health, Natural Medicine: A Comprehensive Manual for Wellness and Self-care*. Boston: Houghton Mifflin Co.

Whitaker, J. and B. Adderly. 1998. *The Pain Relief Breakthrough: The Power of Magnets*. Boston: Little, Brown and Company.

Wildwood, C. 1996. *Aromatherapy: Massage with Essential Oils*. New York: Barnes and Noble Books.

CHAPTER ELEVEN: **The Mind-Body Connection in Children and Adolescents**

Arnold, L. E. 1990. *Childhood Stress*. Somerset, N. J.: John Wiley and Sons.

Arnstein, A. F. T. 1999. Development of the cerebral cortex XIV: Stress impairs prefrontal cortical function. *Journal of the Academy of Child and Adolescent Psychiatry* 38(2):220-2.

Bremne, J. D. and E. Vermetten. 2001. Stress and development: Behavioral and biological consequences. *Developmental Psychopathology* 13(3):473-89.

Brown, J. D. and M. Lawton. 1986. Stress and well-being in adolescence: The moderating role of physical exercise. *Journal of Human Stress* 12(3):125-31.

Dacey, J. S., and L. B. Fiore. 2000. *Your Anxious Child: How Parents and Teachers Can Relieve Anxiety in Children*. Somerset, N. J.: Jossey-Bass.

Depression in Children and Adolescents. Rockville, Md.: National Institutes of Mental Health. NIH publication no. 00-4744.

Haggerty, R. J., L. R. Sherrod, N. Garmezy, and M. Rutter, eds. 1996. *Stress, Risk, and Resilience in Children and Adolescents: Processes, Mechanisms, and Interventions*. Cambridge, U. K.: Cambridge University Press.

In Harm's Way: Suicide in America. Rockville, Md.: National Institutes of Mental Health. NIH publication no. 01-4594.

Keith, C. 1998. Stress in children. *Journal of the Academy of Child and Adolescent Psychiatry* 37:1340.

McCracken, J. B. 1987. *Reducing Stress in Young Children's Lives*. Washington, D. C.: National Association for the Education of Young Children.

McEwen, B. 1999. Development of the cerebral cortex XIII: Stress and brain development II. *Journal of the Academy of Child and Adolescent Psychiatry* 38(1):101-3.

Monk, C. 2001. Stress and mood disorders during pregnancy: Implications for child development. *Psychiatric Quarterly* 72(4):347-57.

Miller, T. W. 1998. *Children of Trauma: Stressful Life Events and Their Effects on Children and Adolescents*. Madison, Conn.: International Universities Press.

Shrier, D. K. 1997. Severe stress and mental disturbance in children. *Journal of the Academy of Child and Adolescent Psychiatry*, 36(8):1154-5.

Teenage Brain: A Work in Progress. Rockville, Md.: National Institutes of Mental Health. NIH publication no. 01-4929.

Westermeyer, J. J. 2000. Severe stress and mental disturbance in children. *American Journal of Psychiatry* 157(2): 295-6.

APPENDIX A: **Time Management and Stress**

A Guide to the Project Management Body of Knowledge (PMBOK Guide). 2004. Newtown Square, Pa.: Project Management Institute.

Buck, M. L., M. D. Lee, S. M. MacDermid, and S. Smith. 2000. Reduced load work and the experience of time among professionals and managers: Implications for personal and organizational life. In *Trends in Organizational Behavior (v. 7)*, eds. C. Cooper and D. Rousseau. New York: John Wiley and Sons.

Covey, S. 1990. *The Seven Habits of Highly Effective People*. New York: Fireside.

Ferris, T. 2007. *The Four-Hour Workweek: Escape 9-5, Live Anywhere, and Join the New Rich*. New York: Crown Publishing Group.

Forster, M. 2006. *Do It Tomorrow and Other Secrets of Time Management*. London, U. K.: Hodder & Stoughton.

Lakein, A. 1973. *How to Get Control of Your Time and Your Life*. New York: P. H. Wyden.

LeFebvre, K. B. 2009. Prioritize and take stock of your life. *ONS Connect* 24(3):20.

Lucchetti, S. 2010. *The Principle of Relevance: The Essential Strategy to Navigate through the Information Age*. Jacksonville, Fla.: RT Publishing.

Macan, T. H. 1994. Time management: Test of a process model. *Journal of Applied Psychology* 79(3):381-91.

Macan, T. H. 1996. Time management training: Effects on time behaviours, attitudes, and job performance. *Journal of Psychology* 130(3):229-36.

Morgenstern, J. 2004. *Time Management from the Inside Out: The Foolproof System for Taking Control of Your Schedule and Your Life (2nd ed.)*. New York: Owl Books.

Nonis, S. A., G. I. Hudson, L. B. Logan, and C. W. Ford. 1998. Influence of perceived control over time on college students' stress and stress-related outcomes. *Research in Higher Education*, 39(5):587-605.

Sandberg, J. 2004. "Though Time-Consuming, To-Do Lists Are a Way of Life". *The Wall Street Journal* Sept. 10.

Seo, E. H. 2009. The relationship of procrastination with a mastery goal versus an avoidance goal. *Social Behaviour and Personality* 37:911-920.

Shanahi, C., R. Weiner, and M. K. Streit. 1993. An investigation of the dispositional nature of the time management construct. *Anxiety, Stress and Coping* 6(3):231-43.